# Comforting Touch in Dementia and End of Life Care

## Take My Hand

Barbara Goldschmidt and Niamh van Meines

*Illustrated by James Goldschmidt*

SINGING
DRAGON

LONDON AND PHILADELPHIA

First published in 2012
by Singing Dragon
an imprint of Jessica Kingsley Publishers
116 Pentonville Road
London N1 9JB, UK
and
400 Market Street, Suite 400
Philadelphia, PA 19106, USA

*www.singingdragon.com*

**Library of Congress Cataloging in Publication Data**
Goldschmidt, Barbara.
  Comforting touch in dementia and end of life care : take my hand / Barbara Goldschmidt and Niamh van Meines ; illustrated by James Goldschmidt.
    p. ; cm.
  Includes bibliographical references and index.
  ISBN 978-1-84819-073-3 (alk. paper)
  1. Touch--Therapeutic use. 2. Terminal care. 3. Dementia. I. Van Meines, Niamh. II. Title.
  [DNLM: 1. Hand. 2. Massage--methods. 3. Dementia--therapy. 4. Terminal Care. 5. Touch. WB 537]
  RZ999.G644 2012
  615.8'52--dc23
                        2011022877

**British Library Cataloguing in Publication Data**
A CIP catalogue record for this book is available from the British Library

ISBN 978 1 84819 073 3
eISBN 978 0 85701 048 3

Printed and bound in Great Britain

# Dedications

To my mothers, Sophie and Regina, for their love and guidance, and my teachers, especially: Jack Gray, for planting the seed; Catherine Shainberg, for bringing the light of imagery; and Jeffrey C. Yuen, whose teachings fell like rain.

*BG*

To Harry and Amber as always, constant, present and supportive.

To all the people who have allowed me to touch their lives from whom I have learned so much.

*NvM*

'Love is survival benefits, bestowed in a creative manner.'

*Ashley Montagu*

# Contents

# Acknowledgments

The inspiration for this book is due in no small part to psychologist Nanette A. Kramer and social worker Janice Dabney, who undertook a search for meaningful ways to engage residents with severe dementia at Cobble Hill Health Center in Brooklyn, New York. That quest led to a research proposal, 'Effects of Specialized Training of Family and Nursing Home Caregivers in the Use of Music and Touch with Nursing Home Residents with Advanced Dementia' that was funded by a New York State Department of Health Dementia Grant in 1996. The administration at Cobble Hill provided a level of support and enthusiasm that made all participants feel a valued part of the team.

Dr. Kramer and Ms. Dabney supervised subsequent opportunities to bring touch into residents' lives. Thanks to the American Massage Therapy Association, a 1998 grant supported an educational outreach so more families of residents could learn the protocol. In 1999, the United Hospital Fund provided a grant for a project called 'Sweet Dreams', which used the protocol to incorporate skilled touch into the bedtime routine. That project had the honor of receiving a best practices award from the American Society of Aging/Brookdale Center on Aging of Hunter College.

Residents were able to continue receiving comforting touch thanks to the Swedish Institute, a college of health sciences in New York City, which sent students from its massage therapy program to work there as part of a supervised internship. A similar opportunity for massage therapists and supervised students was provided by Dr. Russell Portenoy, at Beth Israel's Jacob Perlow Hospice (now MJHS Hospice and Palliative Care Unit).

We are grateful to the following individuals who shared their knowledge, expertise or time to help us create and complete this book: Rocco Caputo, Fred Curtis, Mary Rose Dallal, Jeanne M. Denney, JD Elder, Alexandra Goldschmidt, Rachel Goldschmidt,

Chris Jacob at HeartMath, Jean A. Leone, Diane Rooney, Catherine Shainberg, Pieter Sommen, Rona Weiss and Jeffrey C. Yuen. To all, a heartfelt thank you.

We sincerely appreciate all of the researchers, administrators, and healthcare practitioners who devote their professional lives to providing comfort and quality of life for people with dementia and in hospice care. Family caregivers are a powerful resource; we hope they will find this work useful.

Finally, thanks to the team at Jessica Kingsley Publishers—Lisa Clarke, Emily McClave and Claire Cooper—who recognized the worth of the subject matter and provided the means for bringing it into the world as a book.

# Part 1

# A Sense of Connection

# Chapter 1

# Your Radiant Sea

When someone you love is chronically ill, elderly, or approaching the end of life, you want to spend time with them and you want to be helpful. You might feel overwhelmed with trying to understand the illness, its effect on the person you love, and the treatments he or she is undergoing. Not knowing what to do can add to the stress that you feel; family members often say they feel 'at a loss' about how to play a meaningful role in a relationship they still want to share, despite the changes taking place.

When *New York Times* book critic Anatole Broyard was hospitalized with a chronic illness, he wrote about visitors who looked at him with an 'embarrassed love'. In his column he quoted a therapist who defined embarrassment as 'a radiance that doesn't know what to do with itself'. Broyard wanted a guide that could teach a sick person's family and friends how to make the most of that radiance (Broyard 1990, p.29).

That observation and wish were right on both counts: We *are* radiant, and the energies we emit *can* be beneficial. And while no one would give up the power of modern medicine, the longing for such a connection cannot be fulfilled by technology. This is a power that emanates only from living beings.

The image of a human being as radiant—that is, both particles and waves, matter and energy—is old and new. It has been part of some healing traditions for thousands of years and is now being researched by mainstream medicine. Medical doctors, nurses, homeopaths, naturopaths, acupuncturists, psychologists and bodyworkers—as well as their patients and clients—are among those who have an expanded view of health that includes body, energy, spirit, relationships and the environment. This approach, often referred to as integrative health care, is not only about the integration of different therapies; it also means integrating all aspects of being human. Briefly defined these are:

- *Body*—The physical nature of human beings consists of the tangible aspects of the body, such as organs, glands, blood and genes. These substances can be measured and analyzed.

- *Energy*—The non-physical aspects of the body—such as warmth, breath, sound and magnetism—are less tangible and travel in waves, as do all other energies in the spectrum of life. The vibratory aspects of our surroundings—like sounds, smells and light—will resonate with the energetics of the body and can be an influence on both physical and psychological functions.

- *Spirit*—The quality of what you do comes from the spirit with which you do it. The 'spirit' that is part of the physical body refers to the many dimensions of mind—including conscious and sub-conscious realms, emotions, dreams, memory, projections, purpose and creative inspiration. It is a personal source of spirit, used with a small 's'. When associated with the source of these animating forces it becomes Spirit with a capital 'S'. There are many traditions with rituals and beliefs for approaching Spirit. While these traditions can be very meaningful and comforting for people who are ill or approaching end of life, this text focuses on the personal sense of spirit rooted in the body, without any religious connotation. This personal sense of spirit is especially important when using touch.

These three components constitute the body, and can be used consciously to create changes that are both tangible and vibratory. Their usefulness is fundamental in many traditional practices. Though some of the techniques presented in this book are derived from classical Chinese medicine, acupuncture and acupressure are now used worldwide. A body–energy–spirit system is not only an *Eastern* perspective; it is a view of a living matrix common to all human beings. Its timeless and universal nature are the reasons it continues to be relevant throughout the ages.

Touch is unique because it can influence all three aspects of a person, and depending on intention can place emphasis on one aspect over another. You can choose to use touch on any one of these levels, or all of them; it is up to you. Whichever way you go, it will be an interesting and rewarding experience.

## Sharing your radiance

Touch is the first sense to develop and is a fundamental need throughout our lives (Montagu 1978). When you learn to use touch to communicate, you may discover an alternative to words that can satisfy a deep need. When someone is elderly, chronically ill or approaching end of life, and everyday roles and abilities are lost, caregivers are naturally drawn to non-verbal ways to communicate. They will attach more significance to the flicker of light in the eyes, the rhythm of breath, or the squeeze of one's hand to indicate awareness. With focused touch, you will find that your physical presence and the energy of your love, kindness and compassion can indeed become an important part of communication.

This book is offered as inspiration for caregivers who wish to share touch to provide comfort for a loved one or friend. It presents a hand massage sequence that is grounded in 20 years of practice in both Western and Eastern bodywork traditions. Exercises for increasing awareness and sensitivity are included, since providing therapeutic touch is more than technique. A variety of exercises for cultivating a body–mind approach to touch can be found throughout the book in the boxes identified as 'The inner practice'.

There are also stories about sharing touch, taken from the authors' experiences as a licensed massage therapist and a nurse practitioner working in skilled nursing facilities and hospices. These real-life situations illustrate how the use of touch unfolds at a gradual and individual pace.

Though it can be helpful, touch is not for everyone. Some people have an aversion to touch, for any number of possible reasons. It is an acceptable part of human nature and should be honored. If either you or your receiver is not interested in touch, or if it is not possible due to circumstances, there are other ways to enhance your care. Suggestions for alternative paths you might consider can be found in Chapter 6 'Before You Begin'.

## The hand as a natural choice

Caregivers instinctively hold hands with the person with whom they wish to offer support. The use of touch suggested in Chapter 8, 'A Hand Massage Sequence', takes hand-holding a little further. It focuses on the hands, adding light massage strokes, attention to points on energy pathways, and focused awareness to create a structured way to share touch.

While the hand is a small area of the body, there are many reasons that make it a good choice for caregiver use in sharing touch. Most people feel comfortable touching someone's hand. The hand is usually easy to get to, no undressing is required, and you can apply many of the theories and techniques of massage therapy. Touching the hands makes sense in reinforcing relationship, as hands are an important part of how we communicate. We wave hello, shake hands, and hug. When someone is ill or aging, and the ability to speak, hear or understand words may decline, touch helps you establish a communication that is no longer verbal, but one that is felt.

Because the hands are so sensitive, they are highly receptive to both giving and receiving touch. The skin there contains many receptors for sensory information: pain, cold, heat, touch and pressure. These receptors relay the information with great precision and detail to the brain, which devotes a quarter of all its motor activity to the hand.

The energetic perspective also points to the hand's ability to affect the upper body, especially the head. In classical Chinese medicine, which describes up to 74 pathways (also called meridians) through which energy flows, the meridian points on the hand and fingertips are used to move energy to the eyes, ears, nose and tongue. The fingertip points are particularly important for their potential to communicate with deep aspects of the body–mind referred to as *Shen* or spirit.

# Studying the effects of hand massage

We touch all the time, so how will touch that is 'therapeutic' be different? Do you need special 'powers'? What benefits might you expect? Is it worth a try? Scientific studies are being conducted in increasing numbers to investigate the benefits of touch therapy for various conditions. Most studies indicate positive effects that make using it worthwhile. The touch is sometimes provided by professional massage therapists and sometimes by caregivers with limited training, including family members.

The hand massage presented in this book was created for a study that investigated the use of touch and music therapy for nursing home residents with severe dementia. People who are in nursing homes and hospitals are most at risk for being deprived of radiant human energy, a force that otherwise passes freely between people who care about each other. Physical interactions are often task-oriented, lack meaning on a deeper emotional level, and fail to create a lasting bond between the caregiver and receiver. Furthermore, nursing home residents have less meaningful verbal communication with their caregivers for a number of reasons, which can add to the isolation they experience.

The study gave family members and nursing assistants, the people who spent the most time with residents, the chance to learn touch as an activity that might provide meaning for them. The approach was relatively simple, safe, readily acceptable between genders, and easily adaptable. The primary intention was for the giver to connect, communicate and provide comfort for the receiver. Experiences of many different caregivers have been compressed into stories found in the boxes titled 'When sharing touch'. Each of these illustrates basic principles that can guide the learning process.

Caregivers were taught the massage in two half-day sessions. They then practiced with selected residents during weekly sessions that lasted about two months, during which time they had assistance and support from a trained therapist. At the end of the study, the research showed that residents had an appropriate, significant response to the touch, with increased relaxation, decreased sadness and less agitation (Kramer and Smith 1999). Caregivers found it to be a meaningful activity.

Though this protocol was created for people with dementia, hand massage is used in many kinds of healthcare facilities and has been the focus of a variety of studies. Hand massage has been researched, for instance, for use in palliative care (Osaka *et al.* 2009), for relaxation for the elderly (Harris and Richards 2010), for comfort for nursing home residents (Kolcaba, Schirm and Steiner 2006) and for postoperative pain (Wang and Keck 2004). When it is part of hospice and hospital offerings, comforting touch may be provided by professionals as well as taught to family caregivers.

## Meeting essence with essence

The full benefit of radiant touch involves more than a series of massage strokes or techniques. To make full use of your vibratory nature and to communicate in a wholistic way will involve both your body and mind. Classical Chinese medicine has long recognized this complementary nature of healing by identifying 'outer' and 'inner' medicines.

The outer medicines are part of the science of the body, and include medications and surgery, as well as herbs and acupuncture. They are often provided by professionals. The inner aspect is part of the science of essence, which places importance on a person's thoughts and emotions and ways to purposefully direct them. The Chinese sages referred to these inner practices as 'refinement'. In their eyes, it is what gives meaning to life.

The inner practices are not just for health purposes, but for expanding intelligence that can be used in all aspects of life. They are based on this premise: The mind is more than the brain; a more comprehensive view of the mind includes the whole body and the energetic program that orchestrates it. It has both conscious and below (sub-)conscious activities. Jeffrey C. Yuen, a renowned Taoist teacher of classical Chinese medicine and Dean of the Acupuncture Program at the Swedish Institute in New York City, tells his students that through an inner practice like meditation they can more fully access their awareness to discover their 'fountain of creativity'.

Everyone can experience this connection. A nursing assistant shared an example of how using touch had changed her and the way she worked. At the end of an eight-week training program, she told a story of how she had decided to practice the protocol with her resident in the day room right after lunch. In the middle of their session, some of the other residents started to argue, which led to a brief food fight. But she and her resident had remained an island of calm in the middle of it all. She was impressed at how well she had been able to maintain her focus. 'Why is that?' she asked. 'Is this some kind of meditation?' And then she added, with a little bit of reproach, 'Why isn't this being taught all over the world?'

That question can best be answered with more questions: Who should learn touch? Who will educate caregivers? How will classes and follow-up be funded?

## Caregivers as a community

This book provides a simple and structured way for people to share touch. These may be sons and daughters caring for their ill and declining parents. They may be husbands and wives, nieces and nephews, or parents, providing care for loved ones. Caregivers wear many hats: some of them come to sit, talk and spend time; others may cook, clean, shop and pay the bills. Many of them bathe, turn, feed and clean the people they care for. We hope that the information shared here will inspire them to give new thought to the way they use touch, and the many meanings it can have.

While the focus is on family caregivers, a text like this may also be of interest to nurses and nursing assistants working in healthcare facilities. Perhaps social workers, chaplains and volunteers who visit people at home or in hospitals may have an interest in incorporating touch into a care plan.

Whether they are family or staff, all caregivers keep the ill person company, offer valuable emotional support and create meaningful moments that can never be duplicated. They may be unpaid, and many are underappreciated, but all do it for the love of caring and with kindness in their hearts. There is a great need for the physical, energetic and spiritual contribution that only caregivers can provide.

The use of massage for health care needs is part of a movement towards integrative medicine that began in the 1970s. It was a quest initiated by people who were looking for more natural ways of living. In terms of health, they wanted body–mind approaches that were non-toxic, education about self-care, and tools that would empower them. And it may be the people, not the professionals or politicians, who have to keep the movement going by initiating change.

Almost all of the research being conducted into touch finds positive effects that warrant further study. There are rare adverse reactions or side effects. The cost of implementing touch into a care plan is relatively low, but institutions are often hampered by budgetary constraints in their effort to add this therapy to their services. However, the needs of people for comfort and care cannot wait for bureaucratic approval; they need it now.

Everyone who wants to learn about how to participate in the care of their families should be able to get the education they seek from reliable professionals. Want to bring touch into a residence or skilled care facility? Communicate with the administrators, physician, nursing staff, social worker and psychologist. Maybe you can start by sharing a hand massage with them, to show them what you want to do while providing some stress relief for them at the same time.

What if they give approval, but there is no funding for classes and organized support? Meet other caregivers and pool your resources. Find out about applying for a grant or creating a fundraiser. Lobby for safe, innovative approaches to bring into your situation.

As a caregiver who wants to provide comforting touch, you should not have to feel alone, but should be able to enjoy the input and support of the care management team. As part of an interdisciplinary group, you can bring the value of medicine together with the benefits of your caring heart. This, some people believe, is the act that will lead to the transformation of health care across the globe—the larger radiant sea that all humans share.

# When sharing touch: Begin simply

Ms. F., a certified nursing assistant in a skilled nursing facility for 15 years, was very busy on the geriatric unit, yet, she was caring and energetic enough to volunteer for a research project investigating touch therapy as a way to help residents with severe dementia. Her resident, 'Anna', no longer had voluntary control over her muscles and rarely spoke. Ms. F. did everything for her. Anna's arms, due to contractures, were rigidly held to her chest with her fists tightly clenched. This made the task of dressing and bathing more difficult for her loyal nursing assistant.

At the first training session, Ms. F. learned the gentle massage protocol she would apply to her resident's hands. Ms. F., as enthusiastic as she was to find a way to help Anna, became a bit nervous. She touched Anna throughout the day, yet now she was being asked to touch as if touch alone were going to do something. Did she need to have 'magic' fingers in order for it to have any effect, she wondered. Would she even be able to do a hand massage on fingers so tightly clenched that Ms. F. had to force rolls of cotton into Anna's hands to prevent her nails from breaking through the skin on her palms.

When Ms. F. first learned the protocol, she practiced on a fellow nursing assistant. In the classroom it was easy. Everyone was cooperative and responsive. But she knew it would be different when she worked with her resident.

A licensed massage therapist went to the unit with Ms. F. for her first session. As Ms. F. watched the therapist demonstrate the soothing work, she felt her worry melt away. She realized that there was no magic here, no superhuman demand, none of the tensions associated with doing medical procedures, no false sentiment required. The stroking was simple, and she sensed a kind of pleasure in it, one that her resident might be able to share.

Due to the contractures, Ms. F. started where she could, limiting her touch to Anna's arms and clenched fists. After about three weeks of using focused touch at least two times a week, Ms. F. noticed that Anna's arms were slightly less rigid. What's more, the cotton ball she used to have to force between the fingers and palm now slipped in and out easily. Sometimes it would even fall out during the day, a great surprise to Ms. F.

Soon she was able to extend the stroking all the way down the fingers. Before the end of the three-month research period, Ms. F. was able to lift Anna's arms fully away from her sides. She said getting her dressed was 'no problem' now.

Over time she had been able to extend Anna's fingers one by one. And one day as they were completing their morning routine, Ms. F. took Anna's hand in hers and then Anna raised it to her lips and gave Ms. F.'s hand a kiss. It seemed a fitting gesture of affection and gratitude for the woman she associated with all the comforts of home.

## THE INNER PRACTICE: BODY
### AND BREATH AWARENESS

People who use touch professionally usually make it part of their work to prepare themselves beforehand so they can offer touch with a sense of quiet and calm. They do physical and/or mental exercises to clear the mind of ordinary concerns, a process that may be referred to as 'centering' or 'grounding'. Finding a way to do something similar will enhance the effects of your presence or your comforting touch, at least for the short period of time while you are engaged in doing so.

Suggestions for ways to explore centering are included in most chapters as part of the inner practice of providing touch. If at first you find it hard to feel centered, don't despair; it is a common difficulty. Switching gears and becoming centered may be a challenge, but it is worth the effort.

One of the first suggestions for centering is to focus on physical sensations instead of thoughts. A traditional way to do this is by paying attention to your breath. This is neither a relaxation nor a meditation. It is an observation of your breath and your body, in the moment.

1.  *Assume a comfortable, seated position.* With your hands resting on your lap, breathe out normally, exhaling slowly. It helps to close your eyes so you can focus within.

2.  *As you exhale, let go of any tightness you don't need.* Feel the weight of your body on the chair, letting the chair support you. Inhale.

3.  *Exhale again, slowly.* See the number one, letting all the different parts of yourself become one. Become aware of the flow of your breath, in and out.

4.  *As you continue to breathe with awareness, observe the physical sensations in your body.* Do you feel areas of warmth or coolness? Discomfort anywhere? Tingling or tightness? Don't judge what you feel, just notice it.

5.  *Next, observe the flow of your breath.* Is your breath fast or slow? Does your breath flow in to the level of your throat, your chest, or your abdomen?

6.  *Observe the flow of your thoughts.* How quickly do your thoughts come and go? What is the nature of your thoughts?

7.  *Let any other information from your body come to your awareness.* Breathe out slowly. Open your eyes. Note what you have experienced.

A brief assessment like this can be done before and after giving comforting touch. It may not be easy to do this brief exercise, as it asks you to slow down and most people are used to being continuously active. One student, for instance, reported that he felt nothing when observing his body and breath. But later he admitted that he didn't like doing the exercise because, in his words, 'As soon as I started, I felt hot, my face got red and I wanted to jump up.' Though there was a lot going on, he thought it was not what he was *supposed* to be feeling. He was not objectively observing what he felt.

Recognize sensations that are present, whatever they may be. If there is some discomfort, the next step would be finding a way to address the situation. The agitated student, for instance, could imagine a choppy sea and gradually imagine the waves growing smaller until they become calm, clear waters. Or he could ask himself, 'Where is my source of coolness?' Sometimes people get restless because they are dehydrated, so pay attention to your own needs for food and water.

Because this involves a creative process, there are as many options for response as there are individuals. The Resources section at the back of the book has some suggestions for finding help in learning to embrace subtle sensations as a communication between body and mind. Discovering this link, and acting upon it, provides a deeply felt sense of connection to an inner source of stability and flexibility.

It is a good idea to experience what receiving the touch feels like, so if possible, plan to have someone practice the protocol on you. Do this assessment of the breath and body before and after the practice session, so you can see what changes occur in your own body. Having your own felt sense of what happens will help build your confidence in how to use touch to comfort and connect.

Chapter 2

# Sharing the Benefits of Touch

There is a centuries-old saying in the Eastern healing tradition that 'the medicines that come with the body can extend life' (Cleary 1986, p.117). This may sound esoteric, but modern research confirms that the body constantly produces various substances that regulate physical processes, such as the daily rhythms of sleeping and waking, the stages of development, and healing. Furthermore, studies show that touch can influence some of those inner 'medicines', reducing some and increasing others to alter the body's chemical balance in a positive way.

Brief periods of comforting touch, as little as three minutes, can create calm, reduce anxiety and increase feelings of being loved. Positive touch has been shown to stabilize the heart rate, slow down breathing and enhance the immune system. Changes like these may take place when touch is used by professionals, but research shows that ordinary people—family members or interested friends—are also capable of creating measurable differences in relaxation and pain.

## When touch becomes comforting

You may be touching someone you care for all the time, but you don't necessarily have a therapeutic or comforting effect. That's because everyday touch is often mechanical; it's done without thinking about it, is usually task-oriented and brief. Touch becomes therapeutic or comforting, however, when:

- *It has an intention; you use touch for its own sake and choose specific techniques.* The intention of the touch described in this book is to provide comfort and to invite communication, whether verbal or non-verbal.

- *The unique needs of the receiver are considered.* When working with healthy people, the focus of massage is often areas of muscle pain, stiffness or tightness. Frail populations need a lighter approach, like the touch you would use when applying lotion to the skin. Elderly people appreciate slow, soothing and deliberate movements. People with dementia usually benefit from repetitive, predictable strokes.

- *It is used with awareness; you are aware when you touch and when you stop touching.* By bringing your attention to sensations you feel as you touch—for instance, is the receiver's skin warm or cool, are there areas that are constricted or weak?—you will begin to 'give as a receiver'.

- *It is sustained.* You maintain awareness of your touch and the connection it is making for a period of time, generally from three to 30 minutes. Some part of this time may include non-moving touch, which allows you to sense interactions at the level of the skin, and is a way to let your touch penetrate without having to use pressure. In a study with people with dementia, one group of caregivers was taught a massage protocol (the experimental group) while another group was told to do whatever they considered helpful (the control group). The control group used touch, but it was brief, while the experimental group focused on using touch for 30 minutes. The caregivers using the structured touch had a relaxing effect on the receivers and found it to be a meaningful activity (Kramer and Smith 1999). Purposefully sustaining the touch was a crucial part of its significance for both caregivers and recipients.

With an educated approach and some practice, touch, which is something we use all the time, can have measurable benefits and be a way to amplify a caring intent.

## Physical responses to touch

The yearning for a body–energy–spirit approach to health may have been a part of some people's need throughout history, but it wasn't until the early 1970s that the quest involved so many that it became a movement known as 'wholistic' healing. In addition to recognizing the needs of the whole person, this approach also sought natural remedies and a fundamental understanding of wellness and disease, not just treatment of symptoms. Wholistic practices have been growing in use since then by both individuals and institutions (Eisenberg *et al.* 1993).

The approaches popularized by the interest in wholistic healing—such as massage, acupuncture, imagery, prayer and exercises like yoga and Tai Qi—became known collectively as complementary and alternative medicine (CAM) or integrative medicine. As these therapies grew in popularity, medical researchers took notice and attempted either to verify or disprove benefits.

Touch was never taken seriously until investigators realized what happened to people when they were not touched. The effect of lack of touch in a controlled human population became apparent when healthcare professionals turned their attention to institutionalized infants in the U.S. in the early 1900s. A report in 1915 that looked at children's institutions in ten different cities, found that in most of them every infant under two years of age died. A child's inability to thrive, or *marasmus* as it is medically termed, was a mystery until pediatricians found that infants who were routinely picked up and cuddled survived much better. Based on their findings, several hospital pediatricians instituted a regimen, which became known as mothering in the late 1920s, and the mortality rate fell dramatically (Montagu 1978).

Inspired by this history, Dr. Tiffany Field applied the concept of using touch to premature infants in a study conducted in the late 1980s. At that time, premature infants were isolated and touched very little due to their fragility. Dr. Field's groundbreaking research with premature infants showed that touch, when properly applied, could help them gain weight, grow more rapidly, and get discharged from the hospital earlier than a control group that did not receive massage (Field *et al.* 1986). In 1992, Dr. Field created the Touch Research Institutes at the University of Miami, the first center in the world dedicated to the scientific study and medical application of touch.

The study of the effects of massage is relatively new and has its challenges because massage is not a single 'medicine' but is a broad term that includes many kinds of practices, from acupressure to zone therapy. For the purposes of research, a generally accepted definition of massage describes it as the 'manual manipulation of soft tissue intended to promote health and well-being' (Moyer, Rounds and Hannum 2004, p.4). In this book, the terms 'massage' and 'touch' are both used to refer to the purposeful way of touching described above.

Another challenge in researching massage is the difficulty in 'blinding' a person to the treatment being tested. When a new medicine or medical treatment is being studied, it is considered 'experimental' and is typically compared with a 'control'. For instance, people taking an experimental medication may be compared with people receiving an inactive substance (a placebo). Other controls can be a standard treatment, no treatment or a subject's pre-treatment status. Usually the receiver doesn't know whether he or she is receiving a genuine treatment or the placebo. That may be easy with a pill, but is nearly impossible with a massage therapy treatment.

Many of the early studies of massage, which were limited in funding, are faulted for not being rigorous enough. Research studies typically evaluate an individual's state of being before and after the experimental treatment, comparing data such as heart rate, blood pressure, subjective reports of mood and symptoms, and hormonal effects that can be measured by blood tests. These kinds of studies are expensive, and in the case of massage there is no rewarding 'product' at the end to motivate corporate investors.

Many studies involve small numbers of people, another criticism of early massage studies. That is starting to change as interest grows. As in much other research, there are some conflicting findings. Most studies conclude by suggesting larger and/or more rigorous trials are needed before definitive conclusions can be drawn.

Despite the difficulties, researchers are doing their best to study the effects of massage objectively. While controversy does exist, and alternative methods of conducting valid research are being sought, the emerging results provide some measure of confidence that comforting touch can be beneficial and safe. The most common findings suggest that touch used in a therapeutic way:

- reduces stress and anxiety

- provides comfort and connection

- reduces pain

- improves quality of life

- has benefits for givers.

## Reduces stress and anxiety

One of the most consistent research results is the ability of massage to reduce stress reactions in the body. Dr. Tiffany Field, director of the Touch Research Institutes at the University of Miami School of Medicine, has conducted a number of different studies that show that massage can reduce cortisol, a hormone associated with stress (Field 2000). Researchers looking for an alternative to using blood samples took measurements of a substance in saliva, chromogranin A (CgA), to show that massage could reduce stress (Osaka *et al.* 2009).

One analysis of 37 studies of massage therapy found a course of treatments led to reductions in anxiety and depression similar in magnitude to those of psychotherapy (Moyer, Rounds and Hannum 2004).

A different analysis of nine studies found that a back massage of three minutes resulted in a reduction of anxiety and had some positive effects on participants' cardiovascular function (Labyak and Metzger 1997). When muscles relax, other functions improve, such as the immune system (Mower 1999), and ability to breathe (Wang and Keck 2004). In populations with dementia, a hand massage of 10–15 minutes can increase relaxation (Snyder, Egan and Burns 1995). Even a short period of relaxation can have a great significance, as stress can lower the body's immunity and contribute to the experience of pain (Osaka *et al.* 2009).

In daily life in a nursing home, brief massage interventions can be a potential tool to help calm residents when they are confused or become agitated during routine care activities.

## Provides comfort and connection

Research shows that while touch can *decrease* levels of a stress hormone, it can *increase* levels of another hormone—oxytocin—a neuropeptide associated with feelings of connection and trust (Rapaport, Schettler and Bresee 2010). Most people who are ill or elderly have an increased need for connection. As people age and experience visual and hearing losses, their ability to derive meaning from words or facial expressions is also reduced, resulting in a greater reliance on tactile communication. Unfortunately, the elderly who need it the most are among the most touch deprived in our society (Barnett 1972).

The elderly are sensitive to the quality of touch and what it conveys. When residents of a nursing home watched a video of nurses listening to patients, those nurses who touched a patient's arm while listening to them were seen as being more affectionate and caring (Moore and Gilbert 1995). Touch used with the elderly, including those who are confused, increases interactions like verbal and non-verbal responses, eye contact and more appropriate responses to requests (Vortherms 1991).

## Reduces pain

Another 'inner medicine' that touch seems to stimulate are endorphins, the body's natural pain reliever (Kaada and Torsteinbø

1989). This effect works in concert with other demonstrated benefits of massage—such as decreasing stress, anxiety and depression—to help reduce the perception of pain.

One study used a 20-minute foot and hand massage for postoperative surgical patients whose pain relief from medications was not being adequately met. Following the massage intervention, researchers found significant reductions in both pain intensity and distress, including significant decreases in heart rate and respiratory rate. Authors concluded that foot and hand massage could be a beneficial noninvasive adjunct for patients whose pain is not adequately controlled by medication, and that it could easily be taught to family members, nurses or other personnel (Wang and Keck 2004).

Results suggesting massage can reduce pain have led to its use in palliative care settings. A review of ten trials that looked at massage for alleviating side effects of conventional cancer treatment found that studies suggest massage may have a beneficial effect on physical symptoms such as pain and nausea, though authors considered the research not rigorous enough to draw definitive conclusions (Wilkinson, Barnes and Storey 2008).

A study that compared Swedish massage to simple touch for people with advanced cancer found that both interventions led to improvements in pain intensity and quality of life over time, despite no increases in total analgesic medication use. The researchers reported that a sample of patients who were interviewed after this study indicated that massage provided comfort, time for reflection and a sense of connection to another (Kutner *et al.* 2008).

## Improves quality of life

Quality of life may be hard to define. One psychotherapist at an urban nursing home summed it up as 'Whatever makes someone feel more alive'. Though quality of life may include many subtle elements, one of the important aspects is surely touch.

Even without special massage strokes, touch used with awareness can help improve quality of life by conveying feelings of security and a sense of belonging. Nursing home residents who were frequently touched while receiving medications had a more positive self-esteem than residents who were not touched (Copstead 1980 cited in Moore and Gilbert 1995). When questioned about how they perceived touch used by the nurse, elderly patients felt it should be used for therapeutic purposes in episodes of pain, loneliness and depression (Day 1973 cited in Clement 1987).

## *Has benefits for givers*

By virtue of the shared physical and energetic manipulations, beneficial changes may occur in the giver as well as the receiver. Research has shown that there are physical benefits for caregivers who provide massage. Elderly volunteers who provided massage for infants had a significant reduction of stress hormones and decreased anxiety. Over the three-week period, they also reported a decrease in depression and an improvement in lifestyle changes. (Field 2000)

As people get more involved in their own health care or the care of loved ones, research becomes relevant to everyone as a guide to practices that are safe and effective. Patients and caregivers need reliable education, along with the input of professionals who can provide their insights and experience, as they become part of the integrative care team.

People interested in wholistic health sometimes make the mistake of thinking that because a substance or therapy is 'natural' that it is perfectly safe, or they accept advertising claims at face value. However, complementary and alternative medicine should not be used as self-medication, in place of conventional medicine or without the advice of professionals, because the benefits, possible side effects and interactions with other therapies and treatments may not be known. That includes the recommendations in this book, which do not constitute medical advice nor take the place of physicians' advice in each individual case. (See Chapter 6 'Before You Begin' for cautions and contraindications for massage.)

# The inclusion of self-knowledge

Though research is important, it may never give us all the answers. It cannot yet explain how and why physical changes take place during shared touch. Furthermore, the effects on energy and consciousness will always be completely unique to some extent, and beyond the realm of reason to explain them completely. Some of the answers we need for making our way through the maze of health care choices must come from how well we know our own body and mind, and how much we trust that sense of knowledge.

## WHEN SHARING TOUCH: BE OPEN

The first time Jean offered a session of touch for her mother with severe dementia she did not know what to expect. Since her mother was frail and bedridden, she knew she would proceed gently and slowly, but beyond that she had no preconceived ideas. She was accompanied by a massage therapist who was there to support her interaction. Both would be surprised by the experience they were about to share.

Together they entered the room of Jean's mother, Ms. N., who was lying in bed tightly clenching the border of a blue acrylic blanket. Jean greeted her mother and asked her if she would like some gentle touch. Though she did not produce any distinct words, Ms. N., seeing a stranger in the room, clenched her blanket more tightly and seemed to shrink back into the bed, a response they took as a 'no'. So Jean sat and spoke to her mother quietly.

After a little while, she asked again, and this time Ms. N. seemed to agree to participate with a slight nod of her head, though she still didn't speak any distinct words. Her daughter explained that she would be touching her arms and hands and assured her that nothing she did would hurt.

Since only the top of Ms. N.'s hands were available, Jean began by simply stroking the top of her hand from the wrist to the knuckles.

Her mother watched her with soft, warm eyes. After a few strokes, Ms. N. let go of her blanket, allowing Jean to stroke the full length of her fingers. At that point, she grasped her daughter's fingers and said, 'I'm sad.' The massage therapist explained to Jean that an expression of pent-up feelings during a massage is common, and suggested that Jean assure her mother it was okay to feel sad.

When Jean started to hold the meridian point on the thumb, the massage therapist mentioned that because of its many muscles, the thumb is sometimes referred to as 'the smartest finger'. That made Ms. N., laugh. Surprised by the change of emotion, the massage therapist replied, 'I guess the thumb is also your funny finger' and Ms. N. laughed again, with a mischievous sparkle in her eyes. Near the end of the 30-minute session Ms. N. said, 'I feel like singing' and proceeded to sing a little song.

Having started with no expectations, Jean had been open to responding in the moment. As a result, though the strokes had been slow and gentle, Jean had been challenged to keep up with her mother, as her demeanor moved quickly from withdrawal to one of pleasure and near joy. Jean and the massage therapist were rewarded with a lesson that would be a valuable guide in future sessions: make no assumptions.

# THE INNER PRACTICE:
# WARMING YOUR HANDS

The inner practice is about directing energy. Physical exercises have an inner component when you perform them mindfully—in this case, you keep your thoughts focused on the feelings and sensations in your arms and hands as you perform the movements. The goal is to increase energy and blood flow to the hands, so they will be warm to the touch.

## Hand rubbing

Bring the palms together and rub the hands briskly together, until they feel warm. You will need to wash your hands thoroughly before you share a massage, so washing your hands using warm running water is another way to warm your hands. (See Chapter 8 'A Hand Massage Sequence' for details on hand washing.) You can also rapidly open and close your hands—by making a fist and then extending your fingers—as a way to energize them.

## Arm swinging

This exercise helps to regulate your rhythmic center—the lungs and heart. It has been used through the ages by teachers of Taoism, a philosophy that greatly influenced the development of classical Chinese medicine. They say that if you do it 100 times a day you will live a long life; do it 1000 times a day and you become an immortal!

1. Stand with your feet shoulder-width apart, with the arms hanging loosely by your sides.

2. Your palms face back, fingers relaxed and close together.

3.  Feel your feet planted firmly on the earth; your head lifted slightly towards the heavens. This should create a sense of space in your chest area.

4.  Focus your eyes on a point about ten feet away.

5.  To begin, move your arms backward, and then let them swing up freely in front of you, no higher than shoulder height.

6.  Let your arms drop back and swing forward again, establishing a smooth, continuous swinging rhythm up and back.

## Imagery added

Begin in a standing position; feet shoulder-width apart with your hands at your sides, palms facing your thighs.

1.  Raise your arms up and out to the side so they are about at the level of the shoulder (or wherever you are comfortable) with the palms facing down. As you slowly move your hands back down toward your sides, imagine that your hands are moving through warm water. Bring them to your sides. Breathe out.

2.  Bring your arms up again. This time as you bring your hands down, imagine they are moving through honey. Bring them to your sides and breathe out.

3.  Bring your arms up again. This time, as you bring your hands down, imagine that the tips of your fingers are crayons, leaving trails of color in the space around you. Bring your hands to your sides. Breathe out.

(Exercise used with permission of Catherine Shainberg, Director, School of Images.)

# Chapter 3

# The Body as Particles and Waves

Our radiance as human beings comes from the physical and energetic aspects of the body. When we sense the body as both matter and energy—particles *and* waves—we can begin to understand how a person is affected not only by obvious interactions, but also by more subtle influences like touch, sound, light and even thoughts. This perspective is important in appreciating and embracing our role in integrative health care, because it is these personal energies that are often forgotten or underappreciated in standard medical care.

## We are many energies

We readily accept that we consist of different kinds of matter—skin, fluids, tissues, organs, glands, bones, blood. However, we also embody different types of energy: we emit sounds that can be soft or loud; generate movement of our muscles; maintain a temperature of about 98 degrees Fahrenheit. These energies are audible and tangible.

Other energies within us are silent and invisible. For instance, the electrical charge of our heartbeat emits an electromagnetic frequency that flows through every cell. This may be invisible, but it can be measured by an electrocardiogram, a common practice in medicine.

There is also energy continuously carrying and transferring information within the body. The communication that takes place between cells consists of swift and subtle interactions. 'In the past, we thought the words of the "language of life" were nerve impulses and molecules,' says researcher James Oschman, in his book *Energy Medicine: The Scientific Basis,* 'but we now see that there is a deeper layer of communication underlying these familiar processes. Beneath the relatively slow moving action potentials and billiard ball interaction of molecules lies a much faster and subtle realm of interactions. This dimension is subatomic, energetic, electromagnetic and wave-like in character' (Oschman 2000, p.251). His suggestion that the electromagnetic communication is primary reflects the view in Chinese medicine that the energy system is the blueprint for development, growth and healing; it is not so much that the body has energy, but that energy creates the body.

Think of it this way: look at a seed. If you give a seed the right environment, something will grow from it. But what is inside the seed? Is there a miniature plant? No. There is the genetic code, an energetic formula with the potential, given the right influences, to become a plant.

Something similar happens with humans. There is no miniature baby in the egg or the sperm. When sperm and egg merge, they become one and immediately start to divide. They begin a process called *mitosis,* in which two cells differentiate into all of the varied systems that make up a living being. When we witness this process through a microscope we see only a lot of movement (energy) at work. Scientists describe the process of cell division and differentiation as biology's greatest mystery. Video clips of this process can be readily accessed through the Internet; turn the sound off and just observe what happens.

While all of the energies within the body may not be well understood scientifically, our bodies know exactly what to do with them and how to use them. All the processes of growth, development and repair are orchestrated by our fundamental energy and take place without our conscious knowledge. Anyone who has watched a cut heal has witnessed the energetic program at work. Fortunately, we do not have to consciously think about healing, digesting our food, or maintaining our body temperature. So what *does* orchestrate these activities?

# The movement of energy through the body

All of the major functions in the body—such as respiration, circulation, digestion—have their own system of communication and the energetic aspect is no different. The energetic blueprint is common to all human beings, and most traditional cultures recognize it in some way. Acupuncture, based on the energy system described in Chinese medicine, provides one comprehensive model that is now used around the world.

Classical Chinese medicine, in continuous use for thousands of years, describes up to 74 pathways (also called meridians) through which energy flows. The Chinese word *Qi* (pronounced chee) is usually translated as energy, although the character used to write *Qi* in Chinese reveals that it is more. It is drawn as both a grain of rice and the steam used to cook rice; in other words, it is both matter *and* energy.

Like the rhythm of the heart, *Qi* is thought to be in every cell of the body, flowing up and down the pathways, monitoring needs and orchestrating changes. The therapeutic practices of Chinese medicine are all about moving *Qi*, either slowing it down when it is overactive or stimulating it when sluggish or stuck. Manipulating points—whether with a needle, fingers, or applications of heat—accomplish this. The comforting touch described in this book incorporates meridian points traditionally used for reducing pain and moving energy in the upper body.

Energetic concepts pose a fundamental challenge to Western science. The study of substance is easy and revolves around measurement; the study of energy described by acupuncturists is challenging and has to be measured in ways not currently in use in Western science. Although energetic therapies are gaining popularity and some, like acupuncture, are being investigated at many academic centers, their effectiveness has not yet been validated by the medical community. There is no agreed upon definition for the term 'energy'. How this system works is a bit of a mystery even to the Chinese, although that has not stopped them from making practical use of the idea for over 2500 years.

## Evidence of energetic benefits

Though research on massage is growing quickly, research on the use of meridian points is less common. Studies that involve the use of specific points usually look at *acupressure* (use of pressure on acupuncture points) or *shiatsu,* a Japanese form of bodywork based on the meridian system. Massage, or touch, to meridian points is of interest to researchers, especially those who might be familiar with acupuncture. Benefits for acupressure include:

- decreasing agitation in people with dementia (Yang *et al.* 2007)

- improving quality of sleep for institutionalized residents (Chen *et al.* 1999)

- reduction of neck pain (Matsubara *et al.* 2011)

- reduction of low back pain (Hsieh *et al.* 2006)

- positive changes in health-related behaviors (Long 2008).

The researchers point to some advantages of acupressure: it can be used more frequently than acupuncture, it can be delivered more economically, and it can be taught to patients and caregivers.

People learning to use acupressure often want to know how 'hard' they should press on a point and for how long. One of the few studies that looked at those questions involved people experiencing fatigue from cancer treatments. The study compared a group using points that were considered 'stimulating' with another group using points thought to be 'relaxing'. Participants applied the acupressure to themselves and were told to use enough pressure to experience a 'de qi' response (described as an ache, tenderness, tingling or possibly no sensation). They were to spend three minutes on each point. Results showed:

- Fatigue was reduced in both groups, on the order of 45 percent to 75 percent. Researchers found that fatigue continued to significantly decrease the more acupressure was performed.

- At least four weeks of treatment were needed to achieve significant effects and seven weeks to achieve maximum effect.

- To have maximum effect on fatigue, participants needed to perform a minimum of 21 to 49 acupressure treatments over seven weeks (approximately three times per week to one time per day).

Surprisingly, the group using the 'relaxing' points had a greater reduction in fatigue than the group using the stimulating points (Zick *et al.* 2011).

## An energetic flow

There is some evidence to suggest that the energies created by the body and mind do not stop at the skin, but extend into the space around the body. There are many devices that can measure the sound, heat and electromagnetic waves the body emits. Researchers at the Institute of HeartMath in California have developed a technology that looks at heart rate variability to see what happens to some of those waves when people interact.

HeartMath researchers study the electromagnetic field created by the heart, an effect they say can be measured up to eight to ten feet away from the body (Childre and Martin 2000). They find that one person's heart (and brain) rhythms can have an immediate effect on someone near them. The signal can be transferred not only when subjects are touching, but also when they are only near each other. This leads them to conclude that energy is being communicated, at least in some degree, through a radiant effect (McCraty *et al.* 1998).

HeartMath researchers find a strong interactive effect between the heart and brain. They say that when positive mental states like love or appreciation are held, the heart rate pattern becomes more harmonious. This can set off a cascade of beneficial hormonal changes throughout the body, a process they call 'coherence'. This is an effect that can be shared. For instance, when a baby cries, the waves produced by his or her heart (the heart rate variability rhythm) go into a distressed pattern, with its frequency becoming scattered and disordered. However, when the baby is brought into the mother's coherent pattern, the child's heart pattern will synchronize with it and return to a more harmonious state.

Many people have sensed this kind of communication, intuitively referred to as 'being in sync'. The shared effect of radiant energy is commonly observed in sessions of comforting touch. Massage therapists who work in healthcare settings comment that sometimes when they go into a room a distraught family caregiver may be nervously attending to their sick relative and the distress in the room is tangible. Often at these times, the massage therapist may offer comforting touch to the caregiver. When a caregiver is willing, and starts to let go of anxiety, the atmosphere in the whole room can change, as anxiety is replaced, at least temporarily, by a sense of peace.

While you may use techniques to manipulate the body or direct the energy flow, the most important part of using touch will not be in what you do, but in *how* you do it. This is the quality, or spirit, that you will bring to your shared experience. Tapping into it involves a process of self-discovery that makes touch a unique and interesting exchange every time you use it.

## WHEN SHARING TOUCH: YOU CAN OFFER COMFORT WORDLESSLY

Louis came regularly to the nursing home to visit his mother with dementia. She hardly acknowledged his presence, was often angry and could not sit still; she constantly walked the hallways. She liked fruit, so Louis brought a piece every time he visited. She would sit down to eat it quickly and then start walking again. That was the extent of their relationship.

Louis learned to use comforting touch in a class for caregivers and then went to the ward to try it with his mom. He confessed to the massage therapist who accompanied him that he didn't know if he could do it, because he wasn't used to touching his mother and she no longer seemed to recognize him. However, with some encouragement he agreed to give it a try.

At the first session, when his mother sat down to eat her piece of fruit, Louis was able to do one small gesture before she was up and walking again. But over the course of the next few weeks, he was gradually able to do more of the comforting touch sequence with his mother. On days when she was agitated she might leave but then return again to sit down with him. She eventually sat with him for the full 30-minute sequence. At that point, she even began to stroke her son's hand in return.

That experience was very satisfying to them both, but it was not the end of the story. When his mother later became ill and went to the emergency room, Louis accompanied her. He said that while she was dying, he held her hand the whole time. And because of the experience they had shared previously, he said he felt a strong connection to his mother through their touch. This is a memory he can cherish for the rest of his life.

## THE INNER PRACTICE: GET GROUNDED

Mountain Pose is a way to both center yourself and absorb energy from the environment to help you when you feel depleted. Begin in a standing position.

1. *Place your feet shoulder width apart.* Imagine that your legs form a triangle with the earth as a base. Let your knees relax, so you feel as if your weight is sinking into the earth. Your chin should be parallel to the floor. Close your eyes if you are comfortable doing so, or you can leave them open.

2. *Feel the places on your feet that connect to the earth.* Relax your arms at your sides or you can place your hands, one over the other, just below your navel.

3. *Exhale slowly and with awareness.* Sense and feel that you release any unnecessary tightness and tension as you exhale.

4. *Inhale slowly and with awareness.* Imagine the blue sky and the sun are above you. Your head is drawn slightly upwards, towards the open sky. What happens in your body? Where is your center of gravity?

5. *Sense and feel that you are standing between heaven and earth.* Imagine that you can absorb *Qi* from the earth through the soles of your feet.

6. *Observe your breath as you stand in Mountain Pose for a few moments.* Open your eyes. Notice what you feel in your body.

# Chapter 4

## A Tangible Spirit

You bring spirit into everything you do. Spirit, in the continuum of body–energy–spirit, involves the inner life. This includes conscious and sub-conscious thoughts, perceptions, daydreams, night dreams, memories, emotions, visions, hopes or fears. Alternative terms might be 'consciousness' or 'awareness'. This is another animating factor—along with the physical and energetic aspects—that streams through your body, your day and your life. It also flows out from you into the world, influencing your health, relationships, work and sense of community. Your spirit will determine not only what you do, but *how* you do it.

When using touch, by focusing your awareness along with the focus for physical and energetic contact, you can weave the inner and outer aspects of life together. This creates another layer of meaning and benefit that goes both ways. Your attentiveness is very important, since your use of touch is like a conversation; when you are consciously present the give and take will be more interesting and more meaningful.

### Quality of touch

The quality of your touch will in many ways determine its message. Like any art form, there are elements that you can use to convey your message more clearly. When you want to provide communication and comfort, you will consider these aspects of touch to enhance your intention:

- *Location*—By choosing the hand you limit your focus to an area that is generally considered acceptable to receivers. Touch should always be receiver-centered, allowing them to have control over where and how they are touched. Choosing the hand will emphasize communication, in which the hand plays a large part.

- *Duration*—By spending time on one area, you move from random touch to structured touch, which will reinforce your connection.

- *Tempo*—Your actions will be gentle, slow and repetitive, all of which will work together to convey a sense of trust and encourage relaxation.

- *Rhythm*—You use both movement and stillness, so important to balance and meaning. Think of the sounds and pauses of music; the changing patterns of night and day.

- *Sensations*—As you vary the sensations—from a light, feathery stroke, to soothing strokes, to aware holding at meridian points—you will engage the receiver's attention and interest.

- *Intensity*—Your physical focus is gentle, at the level of applying lotion to the skin. The energetic focus on meridian points involves simply holding the point. Gentleness encourages trust and relaxation. The action of attention and time are more important than pressure.

In addition to these physical and energetic considerations, your focused awareness is another dimension that can be brought into the shared experience.

## Developing a compassionate presence

Responding in a calm or caring way may not come naturally when someone is angry, upset or in pain, especially when it involves a loved one. To avoid reacting with your own anger or upsetness will be a normal challenge that can affect the quality of your touch.

Learning to take a moment to perform an inner practice—whether taking a breath, using imagery or prayer—is important. There are many traditions that teach these methods, which are now being investigated by researchers who want to make them more accessible and understandable.

Meditation is an inner practice now common in hospital-based programs as a way to help both patients and their families in a wide variety of ways. Many studies that show physical and mental benefits, such as lowered blood pressure and stress levels, have led to meditation's increasing use for integrative care. JD Elder, a licensed massage therapist and coordinator of the Massage Therapy Program at the Hertzberg Palliative Care Institute at Mount Sinai Medical Center in New York City, teaches mindfulness meditation as part of his work with patients and their caregivers. 'Through a mindfulness practice, people learn selectively to disregard a lot of the activity that goes on randomly in the brain and just keep refocusing the mind,' Mr. Elder explained. 'The general idea is to keep neutrally observing the mind's activity without getting lost or caught up in it. A lot of mindfulness practice involves taking responsibility for our own minds. If we don't take responsibility for our own minds, and the way we use them, it's like trying to maneuver a boat with no rudder.'

When the giver can focus, it enhances the touch experience for the receiver. Mr. Elder continued:

> I notice sometimes when I teach massage that the practitioner will be focused for about 20 seconds, before they get distracted. I have to remind them to notice that they have gotten distracted and refocus their attention. If they aren't concentrating on what they are doing, they do a disservice to themselves and to the receiver, who isn't getting the full benefit of the practitioner's/giver's energy and attention.
>
> When we do something like a hand massage, in my mind, the idea is to be able to change the way the environment feels for the receiver, through the senses, rather than through thoughts, by creating a calming and soothing sensory experience. The circumstances of one's health,

for example, may not change necessarily but—given the current circumstances in the current moment—the giver and receiver can ideally put aside thoughts such as worry, and focus instead on a quiet activity, such as how nice it feels to have the hand massaged.

Mr. Elder points to the focused use of the mind—using a technique which can be thought of as a time for relaxation—as a behavior that can change the brain and the body.

They've done studies with long-term meditators that show they have less activation in the amygdala—the area of the brain that's more primal and related to fear and aggression—and more cultivation in the areas of the brain related to empathy, compassion and emotional stability. The more we use a synapse, the stronger the connections between the neurons will be. That's how habit develops. The pathways are created by the practices. Therefore, the same thing can happen when we intervene on someone's behalf to help them focus on something other than thinking about their current circumstances, to help them be more in the moment instead of worried about what may happen next; because the truth is, we only have now.

Caregivers may find that providing touch with awareness can be a way to tap into a source of inner wisdom that may not otherwise be accessible. A mindful approach can help foster the self-management they need to carry out the many day-to-day decisions they make and activities they perform. This is at the heart of meditation, which is practiced not so an individual can achieve an idealized state, but as an offering to alleviate suffering for all people. The physical benefits and sense of pleasure that may come along with it are just the 'side effects' of a meditation practice.

Researchers at the Institute of HeartMath study how thoughts and emotions can influence the brain as well as the heart. HeartMath researchers look at heart rate variability, the measure of beat-to-beat changes in the strength and duration of the heartbeat. The heart rate variability is a measure of health and vitality that can decrease with age and stress. HeartMath co-founder and research director Dr. Rollin McCraty says that 'Certain emotions and attitudes deplete our energy reserves, while others renew them. It really gets down to being that simple—learning to have more self-regulation and choice in our emotional diet' (Alexander 2009, p.3). Part of their mission is to teach people to bring thoughts and the body together; to go from a mind-based awareness to a heart-based awareness. Doing so, they say, has benefits for the individual as well as those who are nearby, due to the electromagnetic field of the heart.

HeartMath has developed learning tools that individuals can use to shift their emotional state from mind-based to heart-based when they feel stressed. According to Dr. McCraty, the value of doing so creates a more coherent heart rhythm that 'brings with it more ordered mental and emotional processes... It's a dynamically stable state, out of which sensitivity to another level of information arises' (Alexander 2009, p.4). Some of the exercises are available free from their website (Institute of HeartMath 2011).

## An expanded intelligence

Ancient practitioners of classical Chinese medicine would be very interested in the research going on at the Institute of HeartMath. Among all the organs and glands, the heart is considered the 'emperor' in command of the body and a repository for the spirit. In the practice of acupuncture, reverence for the heart goes beyond its vital role in maintaining cardiovascular health. Practitioners have different words for the various aspects of mind, including *xin*, which is translated as heart/mind. It is responsible for intelligence, wisdom and spiritual transformation.

In order to bring the body and mind together to access an expanded intelligence, whether you take a Western or Eastern approach, you cannot use force. Instead of having goals—even if you think they are of benefit—use of a detached attention is what gets results. Eastern practitioners have long observed this irony of combining effort with non-effort.

To communicate the sum of this experience they use the image of a crane standing on one leg in the water, waiting for a fish to

Comforting Touch in Dementia and End of Life Care

appear. The crane cannot use willpower to make the fish appear. Instead, the crane stands with calm alertness, waiting for the very first appearance of a fish. Then the crane knows what to do in an instant; if it is not paying attention, it misses its opportunity.

This combination of non-action and action illustrates the idea of *contemplation*, a practice that is part of inner development. Through contemplation, you can be helpful and at the same time relaxed. By letting go of goals and turning from words to a felt experience, you will explore the 'spirit' of communication that goes beyond language. This is especially heartening for those working with people who may be less responsive to words; they can still be reached through mindful touch.

Contemplation begins by creating a shift in yourself. If you bring your body, energy and mind together so you can be calmly focused like the standing crane, you will develop the right combination of 'doing' and 'non-doing' that fosters creative responsiveness. The suggestions for inner practice found throughout the book can be used either just before you begin a massage or during a session if you need to refocus. While you are providing touch, you wouldn't stop to meditate or breathe, but would integrate the principles into situations where you are not sure what to do next.

For instance, if you are working with someone with dementia, depending on the stage he or she is in, there may be a sudden mood change. You do not want to use force to rigidly stick to what you are doing, but should take a moment to evaluate what is happening. At that point, you might pause with your hands resting on the receiver's arm or hand and turn to the inner practice by simply breathing out slowly. This returns you to your center, your heart/mind, from which you can observe without judging.

Allow an answer about what to do next to arise from your shared experience; the idea that comes may be surprising, something you might never have thought of consciously. It could be something simple, like turning off the overhead light or changing position. Maybe the receiver just needs some time and your pause allows them to respond in their own unique way. Or your return to your own center will have a calming influence on the heart of the receiver. Sometimes you need only to bring a mindful hand to

50

someone's shoulder to alleviate distress. This is a body–mind way of sharing. Once you can be present with yourself, you can begin to explore your relationship with someone else in a way that keeps you connected to each other, as well as to your intention and sense of compassion.

## The gift of presence

Caregivers face a daunting challenge when encountering the emotions that illness brings up. They say that the most difficult aspect of their role involves social, cognitive and emotional problems, rather than physical symptoms like incontinence (Kilstoff and Chenoweth 1998). Caregivers with the best of intentions can be challenged by receivers who are socially isolated, disruptive to routines at home and sometimes aggressive.

Touch can be a tool for caregivers to turn to for improving communication. Research shows that structured touch reliably brings about a relaxation response and a decrease in anxiety. Focusing on the physical—which is relatively easy—may change a mood or behavior and may be something caregivers can try as a tangible way to help them in their day-to-day struggles.

One study, hoping to encourage the sharing of more positive experiences for those caring for people with dementia, invited family members and staff to take part in the design, development and evaluation of a hand massage. The receivers were people with dementia who lived at home but visited a daycare center. Caregivers were taught a massage protocol of about 10 to 15 minutes, during which time they applied a blend of oils to the surfaces of the fingers, back of the hands and wrists.

After 18 months of sharing hand massage, caregivers reported they had greater coping mechanisms and improved personal relations with their relative, including more time together and more touch in a calm and caring manner. Three of the 16 family caregivers who took part said that the hand treatment calmed relatives who were often angry and helped them deal more effectively with those difficult behaviors. Overall, caregivers considered the interaction a positive way for them to reconnect with their relative (Kilstoff and Chenoweth 1998).

Bringing awareness into your touch will also help you avoid doing it in a rote manner that makes it feel like just another chore. Let go of goals and focus on the interaction you are having with the receiver, feeling the sensations in your fingertips, observing the receiver's reactions, responding in the moment. You do not need to 'try hard'. Should you get distracted, just exhale and return your focus to the few moments you have devoted to touch.

Although practitioners intuitively know they need to let go of effort to achieve a connection, there may now be scientific evidence for this inner shift. James Oschman reports on observations of practitioners and receivers in his book *Energy Medicine: The Scientific Basis*. In a magnetically shielded chamber, a practitioner held his hand close to a receiver while a sophisticated instrument (a SQUID magnetometer) was used to record the biomagnetic field being emitted from the practitioner's hand. When the therapist relaxed into a meditative or centered state, the instrument detected a large increase in the field. Dr. Oschman reports that the field projected by the practitioner's hand was in the same range of frequencies that biomedical researchers find effective for jump starting healing in a variety of soft and hard tissues (Oschman 2000).

Practitioners and receivers can experiment with this phenomenon on their own. See for yourself what happens when you go from an unfocused to a more focused state. Do you sense and feel more acutely? Is there more energy—e.g. warmth, tingling or pulsing—in your hands? Can the receiver, if they can give feedback, detect a change? This can add another dimension of interest to your exchange.

## A creative leap

The techniques of comforting touch described in the following chapters are not an absolute formula, but a framework to help you focus and begin your practice. It is much like playing a musical instrument or learning to dance. At first, practice is stiff and self-conscious. But when technique becomes automatic, you start to move freely, losing self-consciousness and focusing on the expressions taking place. You discover something new, immediate, meaningful, a way to tap into your 'fountain of creativity'.

Dr. Frederick Leboyer says in his book about infant massage that

> In any art…there is a technique. Which one must learn. Technique and learning take time. But once this technique is mastered, the artist moves beyond it. And beyond time. You touch something in yourself. Or rather, something starts expressing itself in you. Puzzle? Paradox? It is the secret, the mystery of all art. Art, which enables you to touch the absolute. With your very human hands. (Leboyer 1976, p.119)

As you touch, you connect not only to someone else, but to something meaningful within yourself. When you want to help someone you care for, you can prepare by getting clearance from their medical team, looking at research, and having techniques to guide you. All are helpful, but to find your own answers and gain a sense of authority you can tap into your direct experience of the body. The more you learn about the body and how it works, the greater your involvement will be in the rhythms of life and the laws of nature. Only awareness and practice, not the force of your will-power or a gift with words, will reveal the way. It will lead you to the answers that are in your heart.

## When sharing touch:
## Make no effort

Irene learned how to develop and trust an inner sense of guidance when she practiced using comforting touch with her husband Joseph who was a resident in long-term care. Joseph usually sat in a recliner at the nursing home with his eyes closed and his jaw slack. When he did open his eyes, they were usually clouded and unseeing. He never spoke a word.

After her first time sharing touch with Joseph, Irene noticed a small change. 'After the touch session, he went with the aide to take a shower,' Irene recalled. 'When he came back into the room, he looked over at me and when he saw me, a tear rolled down his cheek.' Irene herself started to cry at this description. 'It was the first time he has responded to me since he's been here, about five years now.'

Irene continued to practice comforting touch with Joseph at every visit. During one session Irene began the gentle strokes down Joseph's arm, gliding over the bumps and hollows that flesh and bone create. Irene sat in a chair alongside her husband and massaged the palm, the back of the hand and the fingers. When Irene started to hold the points at the fingertips, Joseph opened his eyes and looked at Irene and seemed to pull his hand away. At first Irene wondered if Joseph was resisting. She paused to see if she could figure out what Joseph was trying to 'say'. Then, quietly and assuredly, she felt, 'Oh, he wants a pillow.' Irene took a pillow from Joseph's bed and placed it behind his head. He relaxed into it and closed his eyes again.

Then Joseph opened his eyes again and they looked different, with a new quality of being lit, of urgency, of struggle. He focused keenly on Irene, tightly holding her hand and pulling her closer. Irene began talking animatedly to him, telling him how people ask about him, what their children were doing, and what was going on in her own life. Something had changed.

It felt as if a strong current between them had been turned on, flowing back and forth and at the same time expanding into a radiant circle around them. It was a tangible thing, which felt both emotional and personal. Such a weaving of energy is an example of human bonding, something that takes place when people share soothing words, prolonged eye contact and comforting touch.

The shared radiant effect of an event like this is described beautifully by humanist Joseph Chilton Pearce, whose observations of the bonding that takes place at birth bear an uncanny resemblance to what had happened between Irene and Joseph. Mr. Pearce, describing the first hour after birth, says that the bond 'is established in strange, mysterious and unfathomable ways. Anyone else around literally gets caught in the magnetic fields of attraction weaving back and forth' (Pearce 1980, p.98). As love unfolds, the heart exudes its power, which can be felt within the room.

# THE INNER PRACTICE: MINDFULNESS MADE SIMPLE

As part of the Palliative Care Institute at Mount Sinai Medical Center, JD Elder teaches this simple meditation technique to patients and their families to help them relax the mind, the body and its systems.

1.  Begin by placing yourself in a comfortable position, either sitting or lying down.

2.  Close your eyes, notice the activity of your mind. What are you thinking? How quickly do your thoughts change? What is the nature of your thoughts?

3.  Throughout the practice time commit to a non-judgmental attitude.

4.  Bring your attention to your breath, its flowing in and flowing out.

5.  Keep returning your focus to your breath.

6.  Allow thoughts to pass through your mind with awareness (mindfulness). Just notice them without engaging them.

7.  When you notice you get distracted by thinking or judging, bring your attention back to the breath, maintaining the non-judgmental attitude.

8.  Practice from one to 20 minutes.

This practice can be done on a daily basis.
(Used with permission of JD Elder.)

# *Part 2*

# Focusing Your Touch

# Chapter 5

# Physical and Energetic Qualities of the Hand

There was a time when almost everyone worked with their hands. Human beings used to build their own shelters, raise their own food, and attend births and deaths. Today, many of us grow up and work in jobs focused more on virtual reality than on fulfilling basic needs; we depend on our intellect instead of our body. Many people, however, want a way to return to 'nature'; it is a yearning that has fueled new interest in organic food, the environment and wholistic health. Using your hands to help alleviate anxiety, confusion or pain can be a way to return to the basics of direct care for someone you love.

The hands are exceptional areas of the body for using touch in a meaningful way and can provide significant value and effectiveness not only for the receiver, but for a person giving and sharing the experience as well. There are a number of reasons touch applied to the hands is a good choice for caregivers looking to provide comfort and connection, especially for receivers who may be elderly, have dementia, or are approaching end of life.

## Acceptance and ease

For almost every population, the hands are usually accessible. Massaging the hands requires no undressing and is generally a well-accepted place to touch between genders. The hand is a small area to which you can apply the basic strokes of massage—gliding, pressure and holding—rather safely. The intervention does not have to be difficult or lengthy; by touching the hand thoughtfully for only a few minutes it is possible to have a positive influence on many physical and mental processes.

## The hands as communicators

Trying to speak to someone who may no longer understand words, or be able to respond to them can be frustrating. However, you can bypass the intellect and use an earlier form of communication—the language of touch. For a touch therapy intervention that focuses on communication, turning to the hand makes sense for a number of reasons. The hands reinforce relationship, as they are an important part of how we communicate: we wave hello, shake hands, write with our hands, and use them to hug. When you use your hands to touch mindfully, you bring this same impulse to communicate. When someone experiences visual and hearing losses that may reduce their ability to derive meaning from a smile or nod, or what is said, touch can be a significant way to convey meaning.

Scientists studying the ability of touch to express emotion found that blindfolded participants could quickly and reliably detect the emotion a giver was conveying. Participants were divided into groups that would either touch or be touched. Those providing the touch were told to wordlessly communicate one of six emotions: anger, fear, disgust, love, gratitude or sympathy. Receivers put their bare arm—from the elbow to the end of the hand—through a curtain so they could not see the sender. The receivers were able to accurately determine the emotion being conveyed 48 to 83 percent of the time (Hertenstein *et al.* 2006).

In a follow-up study, the givers were allowed to touch wherever they felt it appropriate and two more emotions—happiness and sadness—were included. Again, those receiving touch were able to accurately determine the emotion being conveyed 50 to 70 percent of the time, much higher than the 11 percent expected by chance and comparable to rates seen in studies of verbal or facial emotion (Hertenstein *et al.* 2009).

Matthew J. Hertenstein, who led the research, said the results had strong implications for the power of touch. 'Most touches were only about five seconds,' he said in a *New York Times* interview 'but in these fleeting moments, we're capable of communicating distinct emotions, just as we are with the face. This is a sophisticated differential signaling system that we haven't previously known about' (Bakalar 2009).

## Studies show hand massage is effective

Massage to the hands (and in some cases to the hands and feet) has been used in a number of research projects. Briefly, some of the relevant, positive findings on hand massage show that it:

- will be acceptable to most receivers

- alleviates stress for patients

- enhances relaxation

- reduces anxiety and lowers blood pressure

- provides a wholistic sense of comfort

- helps to reduce pain.

### *Will be acceptable to most receivers*

Nursing home residents feel comfortable having the arm and hand touched, while touching the face is perceived as a more intimate contact (Moore and Gilbert 1995). Touch is experienced as positive when it is appropriate to the situation and does not impose greater intimacy than desired (Hollinger and Buschmann 1993). While the majority of people accept touch readily, a small percentage may prefer not to be touched, so individual attitudes should always be taken into consideration and alternatives considered if necessary (see Chapter 6 'Before You Begin').

## Alleviates stress for patients

A five-minute massage to the lower arm and hand was provided for people hospitalized in a palliative care unit of a cancer center in Japan. To determine stress levels, researchers measured changes in saliva (salivary CgA) and through a brief questionnaire. They found a significant improvement after the brief hand massage and concluded that 'therapies such as massage could be valuable non-pharmacological treatments to reduce the physical symptoms of patients' (Osaka *et al.* 2009, p.984). They pointed out that for terminally ill people, even a short period of distress can have a great significance, and that caregivers—including family members—who were able to give a simple hand massage could help to relieve the stress of patients (Osaka *et al.* 2009).

## Enhances relaxation

In a review of 21 studies that looked at back massage and hand massage for older people, all showed statistically significant improvements on physiological or psychological indicators of relaxation. The most common protocols were three minutes for back massage and ten minutes for hand massage, which showed a consistent reduction in verbal aggression in persons with dementia (Harris and Richards 2010).

A study that compared hand massage, therapeutic touch and presence to produce relaxation and reduce agitation in residents of an Alzheimer's care unit found greater increases in relaxation for the group receiving hand massage (Synder *et al.* 1995). Using the hand massage protocol took about ten minutes. Researchers suggested that an intervention like hand massage should be considered for use before initiating care activities or transitions that tend to precipitate agitation in people with dementia.

### Reduces anxiety and lowers blood pressure

Prior to cataract surgery, patients received a five-minute hand massage. After the massage, there was a reduction in anxiety levels, systolic and diastolic blood pressures and pulse rate. The massage also reduced levels of epinephrine and norepinephrine, hormones associated with stress, while the hormone levels increased in the control group who received routine care (Kim *et al.* 2001). Even the simple act of hand-holding for patients awaiting surgery was shown to be an effective intervention for alleviating anxiety (Oh and Park 2004).

### Provides a wholistic sense of comfort

Nursing home residents were divided into either a treatment group, which received a hand massage six times over a five-week period, or a control group that received usual care. The technique took five to eight minutes for each hand. A significant difference in comfort was found within the hand massage group within two and a half weeks; after that, however, both groups showed improvement. 'Wholistic comfort' was defined as 'the immediate state of feeling relief, ease, and transcendence' (Kolcaba *et al.* 2006, p.85).

### Helps to reduce pain

One study looked at the use of a 20-minute foot and hand massage for patients who had undergone surgery and had received pain medication but were still reporting discomfort. The foot and hand massage significantly reduced both pain intensity and distress resulting from incisional pain on the first postoperative day. Researchers concluded that massage could be a beneficial non-invasive pain management strategy for patients whose pain is not adequately controlled by medication, and that the skills could 'easily be taught to family members' and healthcare personnel (Wang and Keck 2004, p.64).

## Sensitivity and the brain

The hand is a small, but complex area that is a great example of the body's amazing design. Though all hands share common characteristics, each person's hand will be as distinctive as the whirling pattern of its fingerprints.

An underlying layer of fat and connective tissue, the fascia, is anchored to the bones to prevent the skin on the palms from sliding around like a glove. The skin on the palms is unique compared to other areas of the body because of its tough, yet sensitive, composition. When you touch with your fingers, the contact with the environment sends an immediate signal to the brain, which explains why the skin is considered an external part of the nervous system. Forty-eight nerves serve the muscles, tendons and skin of the hands, with 24 of them being sensory nerves responsible for discerning different types of touch.

Within the skin, there are many receptors that receive five types of sensory information: pain, cold, heat, touch and pressure. These receptors relay the information with great precision and detail to the brain for interpretation. Tactile stimulation derived from receptors located in the skin is an essential part of development for animals, as well as for humans, and remains a need for most people throughout their lives.

While all areas of the body have corresponding sensory areas in the brain—for instance, there is an area for the arm, the shoulder, the leg—the size of these areas pale in comparison to the amount of cerebral cortex devoted to discerning sensations in the fingers. Of these, the thumb occupies a slightly larger area, being the digit with the most muscles and sensory receptors (Gray 1977; Montagu 1978).

## Meridian points and their effects

Another reason for choosing the hand for massage involves the energetics of the meridian system of acupuncture. There are many meridian points on the hands that can be useful for caregivers who would like to help with easing pain, anxiety or nausea for a receiver. Touching a point has a local effect on the immediate area and will also affect the whole meridian. This means that the points on the hand can be used for both local and distal effects.

A local effect means that the massage creates changes in the immediate area you are touching. Since working with energy has normalizing effects, it can help fingers that may be flaccid as well as those that may be strongly contracted. The points can be used for reducing pain and stiffness in the fingers. Nursing assistants in one facility found that hand massage helped residents with dementia who had contractures to open their fingers, making daily tasks like dressing easier.

A distal effect means working on a point creates changes to the distant end of the pathway. For instance, points on the fingertips have a strong influence on the head and are suggested as a way to 'open the orifices', that is, to send energy to the eyes, ears, nose and tongue. They are said to be important for alleviating depression and anxiety, and for calming the spirit.

There is a saying that 'the eyes are the windows of the soul' and practitioners of Chinese medicine believe something similar about glimpsing spirit through the eyes. When working with people who are non-verbal due to dementia, the eyes sometimes do seem to open like a 'window'. At those moments, as a caregiver holds points on a resident's fingertips, there may be a moment of change, when a recipient who had been disoriented or sleepy suddenly turns to make brief, intense eye contact.

Those moments offer a strong sense of presence, and what feels like an undulating energetic charge. We can only speculate about this inner state, as it is purely subjective and cannot be measured. Some people believe it may go beyond spirit with a small 's' and involve Spirit, that which is connected to a greater presence. The tradition of classical Chinese medicine recognizes Spirit (or *Shen*), as an animating source of life. While some people may initially feel that working with the elderly or dying might be depressing, this concern evaporates if you experience this uniquely personal, yet universal, presence.

Meridian points can also have a general effect. A new Integrative Therapies Program for children and adolescents in Pediatric

Hematology/Oncology at St. Joseph's Children's Hospital in Paterson, New Jersey, is investigating the use of a single meridian point, Large Intestine 4, which is located on the hand. Diane Rooney, a licensed acupuncturist, has been part of the start-up of the new program during the last year and a half. She explained:

> We are doing a research project on acupressure for sickle cell anemia pain crisis. Sickle cell anemia is a lifelong disease in which the red blood cells—which are normally donut shaped with a scooped out middle that make it easy for them to squeeze through blood vessels—turn into a sickle shape or quarter moon shape. Instead of moving through the bloodstream easily, these sickle cells can get jammed at the blood vessels and deprive the body's tissues and organs of the oxygen they need to stay healthy. This causes excruciating pain.

> The researchers place a small suction cup on the meridian point on the hand for about 20 minutes. The cup uses suction for negative stimulation and a small magnet presses down to give positive stimulation. Following the treatment we measure morphine use for 24 hours to see if the children need to use as much morphine, or as often.

As part of the program, Ms. Rooney shows parents how to locate and massage the point so they can continue the treatment at home.

## Key meridian points on the hand

If you look at the hand energetically, you begin to understand why it feels so good to hold hands with someone you love, why a parent's touch can be so comforting, and even why a baby sucks its thumb. The following points, identified by meridian name and number, are used in the hand massage sequence. Descriptions include the location of the point and a few of its actions. Some are particularly useful for a population that is elderly or in cognitive decline.

## Large Intestine (LI) 4

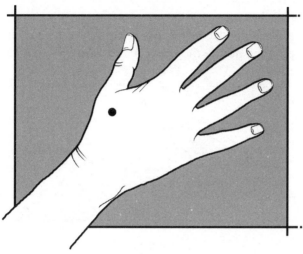

Figure 5.1

**Location:** This point can be found in a depression between the thumb and index finger when you stretch your fingers apart, or at the top of the 'hill' that appears if you bring your fingers together.

**Name:** All meridian points also have traditional names which help to identify either their location or function. This point is called 'Adjoining Valley' because the point is in a 'valley' formed when the thumb and index fingers are stretched apart. Among practitioners it is commonly referred to as 'the Great Eliminator' due to its ability to release pain, anxiety and acute conditions.

**Benefits:** LI 4 is an important point for elimination. It is said to alleviate pain and relax the muscles. It can regulate the large intestine, whether there is constipation or diarrhea. It benefits the tongue (alleviates tongue stiffness), opens and brightens the eyes, clears the nose and quiets the spirit. It is traditionally taught as a general wellness point, and for an acute problem in the upper body, such as a headache, first sign of a cold, or a stuffed nose.

*Important caution: Do not use this point with a pregnant woman because it is associated with the strong downward flow of energy and can stimulate uterine contractions. It is a point used to promote delivery during labor.*

## *Small Intestine (SI) 3*

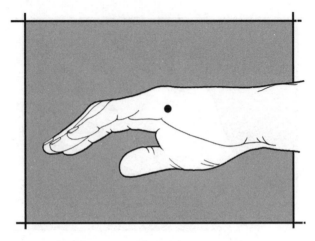

*Figure 5.2*

**Location:** If you make a loose fist, the point is in the depression just behind the knuckle of the pinky finger, at the border of the light and dark skin.

**Name:** This point's Chinese name means 'Back Stream' because of its association with releasing the back and relaxing the muscles, especially in the upper back and neck.

**Benefits:** This point is indicated for acute muscular symptoms of the upper back and neck, such as stiff neck, headache or backaches. It can be used for hypertonicity of the fingers and arms. It is indicated for loss of the voice after a stroke. On a mental level, it is said to calm the mind and aid dream disturbed sleep. By helping energy to flow more freely up the back to the brain, this point is sometimes used—either alone or in combination with other points—to give support to someone facing difficulties (Maciocia 1989).

## Triple Warmer (TW) 4

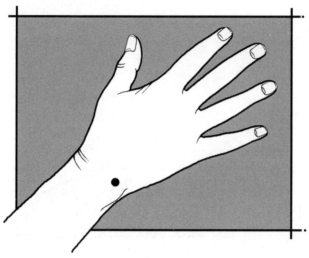

*Figure 5.3*

**Location:** With the palm facing down, trace a line from between the fourth and fifth fingers up to the wrist crease. The point is located in a depression just in front of the bony protuberance.

**Name:** Its name, 'Yang Pool', refers to its importance as a source point for tapping into original *Qi.*

**Benefits:** This point is used to relax muscles and is important for increasing energy. Its use is recommended 'in all chronic disease when the kidneys have become deficient and the person's energy is greatly weakened' (Maciocia 1989, p.439).

## Pericardium (PC) 6

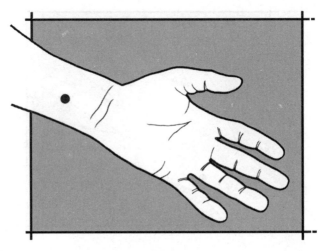

*Figure 5.4*

**Location:** On the inside of the lower arm, about two inches above the wrist crease, between the tendons (of palmaris longus and flexor carpi radialis muscles).

**Name:** The name 'Inner Pass' or 'Inner Border Gate' refers to the point's location on the inner arm, and its connection to a deeper channel.

**Benefits:** This point is said to calm the spirit and clear the chest and brain. Its usefulness in redirecting rebellious stomach *Qi* downward has made it a point commonly used for nausea. A number of studies seeking ways to alleviate nausea have looked at the use of acupressure and acupuncture on this point and found it to be beneficial during postoperative care and chemotherapy, though better designed studies and larger trials are often cited as a need (Chao *et al.* 2009).

## Pericardium (PC) 8

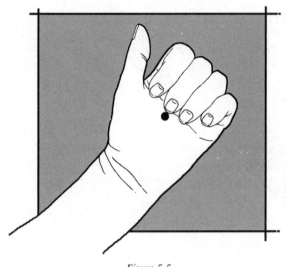

*Figure 5.5*

**Location:** To help find the point in the center of the palm, make a loose fist so the fingertips rest on the palm. The tip of the middle finger will touch PC 8.

**Name:** The point's name, 'Palace of Labor' points to its usefulness after any kind of extended effort.

**Benefits:** This is one of nine points for restoring energy. It is used to restore consciousness and calm the mind. For local effects it can help reduce stiffness of the fingers.

## *Fingertips*

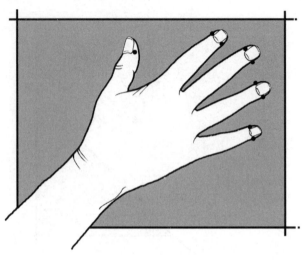

*Figure 5.6*

**Location:** Most fingertip points are at the base of the nail. For ease of use, hold the receiver's finger at either side of the nail (at the points shown) between your thumb and index finger.

**Benefits:** The points on the fingertips are significant because they are where meridians begin or end. Because of that, they can strongly affect the flow of the pathways up or down the arm. All points at the fingertips are said to affect the head and brain, and are indicated for calming the spirit and clearing 'vexation'. In a nursing home or hospital, vexation could be seen as disruptive behavior, agitation around certain activities, or depression.

Points on the fingers can also be used locally to reduce pain, stiffness or tremors in the fingers. In particular, points on fingertips have these effects:

- Little finger benefits the eyes. Additionally, is indicated for 'quivering from the cold' (Ellis, Wiseman and Boss 1991, p.177), which might be useful with an elderly population. (Points at the finger tip are Small Intestine 1, on the outer side of the nail bed and Heart 9, on the inner side of the nail bed.)

- Ring finger benefits the ears and tongue, aids in relaxation. (Point at the finger tip is Triple Warmer 1.)

- Middle finger benefits the tongue. (Point at the finger tip is Pericardium 9.)

- Index finger benefits the ears and moistens the throat. (Point on the fingertip is Large Intestine 1.)

- Thumb calms the spirit, alleviates anxiety and relieves pain. A baby intuitively knows what he or she is doing when sucking its thumb. The baby cries when it's hungry, but will suck its thumb to stimulate this point as a self-soothing measure. (Point on the thumbtip is Lung 11.)

## Spend time at a point

Newcomers to touch always ask, 'How hard should I press?' You will have your answer by looking at who you are working with. The elderly and children do not need, nor do they like, deep pressure. But you do not have to press 'hard' to have a beneficial effect. Pressure is an 'outer' effect. When working from an 'inner' perspective there is very little effort. A more satisfying response comes from trust and the ability to focus, rather than from physical effort.

Like the crane standing on one leg waiting for a fish to appear, when the moment arises you will know what to do. To begin with, just hold a point and become aware of what you sense and feel there. Is it warm, cool, tight or soft? As you hold it, does it change? Which point seems to 'want' to be held longer, or again? Let your senses guide you. See with your fingers; feel with your eyes.

Comforting touch consists of both movement and stillness; they are necessary complements for a harmonious effect. Think of the importance of the pause in music or the restfulness of night after a busy day. When you use touch, movement is the more conscious (yang) expression of care, while stillness offers support and is more sub-conscious (yin) in nature. They will have different effects, both with value.

A class participant illustrated how important connected stillness can be. 'Last week the instructor demonstrated the technique on me,' he said. 'She paused in the lesson to address the class, and while she did, she rested her hands on my shoulders. During the week, whenever I felt stressed, I remembered her hands on my shoulders and I completely relaxed.' This is one of those felt memories that can last for a long time.

Another question that comes up is, 'How long should I hold the point?' A general guideline is anywhere from a minute to three minutes. Researchers who studied the use of acupressure to help people experiencing fatigue from chemotherapy found that working with each of the points in a protocol for about three minutes had a significant effect. Participants applied the acupressure for themselves and were told to engage with the point until they felt a *Qi* response, which could be identified as tingling, warmth, or possibly nothing (Zick *et al.* 2011). They used timers; you should use your felt sense of what is right in the moment for you and your receiver.

People are fond of saying they 'have no time' to do anything, and here is an opportunity to engage in an activity that does not take much time. However, you may be surprised at how long a minute may seem when you are focused. It's as if time slows down. An expanded sense of time is something that may benefit you, especially if it is a real change from the usual stresses of always feeling rushed.

## Your radiant hand

Remember that your hands in general are a source of radiating energies—warmth, movement, electromagnetism and *Qi*. As discussed in Chapter 4, the focused practice of touch can change the energies that emanate from your hands, enhancing their frequency and amplitude (strength) to result in a more penetrating effect. The body–energy–spirit dynamic is an important part of that equation, with power being generated not from greater technical skill, but from greater compassion.

## WHEN SHARING TOUCH:
## SOMETIMES LESS IS MORE

After an instructional session, Mary was eager to try the hand massage protocol on her grandmother. Ms. T. was a resident in the dementia ward who was bedridden and no longer verbal. There was one peculiar and disturbing behavior that Mary hoped to influence. While Ms. T. was lying in bed, she would raise her head up off the pillow and hold it there. If another pillow were placed under her head, she would eventually raise her head up from that one also. This was distressing to watch, as one could easily imagine the tension created in her neck.

Mary went to the nursing home unit with the massage therapist to practice. Her grandmother was lying in bed, with her head raised up from the pillow. Mary looked anxiously at her grandmother. The therapist encouraged Mary to briefly center herself and assume a neutral state of mind that focused on interaction rather than outcome.

Ms. T.'s arms and hands were easily accessible, so Mary began with some gentle stroking down the arm to bring awareness to the hand. She followed with massage strokes to the hand and fingers. Then, encouraged by the therapist, she focused on holding the Small Intestine 3 point, located on the pinky side of the hand. This point, Back Stream, is said to help the energy flow in the back, especially the upper back and neck. Mary held the point calmly as she watched her grandmother.

After a few minutes, Ms. T. began to relax, allowing her head to go down onto the pillow. Mary smiled and looked over at the massage therapist, who guided her to return her

75

to the shared moment. Excitement, even if it is 'positive', can take you out of the moment and disrupt the flow of energy.

Ms. T.'s head came up again, but only for a short while, and then returned to the pillow. She rested that way for a while until her roommate's family entered the space noisily, at which point she stiffened again. But her granddaughter persevered and eventually Ms. T. settled back down and seemed to go to sleep. Mary was happy to have a tool to help her grandmother's distress and said she would continue to massage her hands whenever she was visiting.

## THE INNER PRACTICE: SCAN THE SKIN

You can practice this on yourself, but it will be more instructive if you try it on another person who can give you feedback. Place your hand, suspended in the air, just above the level of the skin surface, over an easily accessible area such as an arm, the back or a leg. Slowly float your palm above the level of the skin, without touching the body.

As you do so, imagine that the pores are like air shafts, emitting currents of varying qualities, such as warmth, coolness, tingling or pulsing. This is the energy at the surface of the body, which brings warmth to the muscles and skin and provides the resources for movement. When someone has an acute illness like the flu, some surface energy is diverted to deeper layers to protect the core, resulting in muscle aches and weakness. Who hasn't experienced this? When the illness is resolved, and energy returns more fully, muscle function returns to normal.

As you scan the area, pay close attention to any variations in the sensations you feel. Is there an area you feel drawn to more than others? Go to that area and focus on the sensations there for a few moments. See if any changes occur.

You might ask the receiver what they feel in that area and how they perceive what happens as you hold your hands above it. Then, with the receiver's permission, place your hands on the body at that area; again, observe what you sense and feel as you let your hands relax and hold the area. Ask the receiver about his or her experience.

# Chapter 6

# Before You Begin

## *Observing Best Practices*

As human beings and caregivers we soon learn that there is no perfect health, no one answer, and no magic therapy that can be used for everything and everyone. Everything we do has benefits and risks. As gentle as it is, and as beneficial as it may be, massage must always be used with caution. In some instances, offering massage may not be the best choice at all given the receiver's state of health or current symptoms.

Some people turn to complementary and alternative therapies— such as herbs and supplements—and use them on their own. Sometimes they do so without knowledge of the therapy or treatment's efficacy. There is often no professional assessment of physical, energetic or psychological functioning from practitioners or trained people knowledgeable about the therapy or treatment. But most important to an integrative approach is remembering not to focus only on symptoms, but to address the individual body-energy-spirit. Because that is where the source of healing resides.

In order to move from being a passive receiver of health care to one who can be involved requires some education and training. Information from reliable sources is one part of it. Risks and benefits of any treatment should be considered. The right mix of intention, knowledge, professional guidance, collaboration, intuition, respect and practical experience is needed to bring all of the elements together for the creation of effective integrative care.

The following guidelines offer important insights and guidance about using massage therapy as part of an integrative care plan. The material comes from the perspective of professionals in the field, and is aimed at providing a safe and effective massage. Medical professionals are guided by research, standards of care and practice protocols. Having said that, the framework for offering effective treatment should be tailored to individual needs with standards of care in mind. Earlier chapters provided information culled from academic and medical research about the benefits of touch. The following are the standards of care that include the cautions you should be familiar with before you begin to use massage.

## Standards of care

The use of touch described in this book is aimed at providing comforting touch. If the receiver is elderly, frail or ill, the first step in using the techniques that follow is consulting with the medical professionals in charge of the care plan. All of the people in studies and in experiences described in this book had medical clearance before receiving any massage or touch. *This is a very important step that ensures that massage is provided appropriately, taking into account the medical conditions and treatments that are relevant to providing comfort care.*

Integrative medicine expands the circle of care—and includes family, friends, patients, doctors, nurses and integrative practitioners like massage therapists—in the process of health, healing and providing optimal quality of life. As you become part of the integrative team, you should obtain professional guidance and observe standards of care. There are a number of factors to be considered when offering comforting massage to people who are receiving various treatments, medications and have symptoms that affect their daily lives. There is no need to feel alone or to proceed without support and guidance. Members of the healthcare team often work closely together to identify the goals of care, create strategies for delivering care and assemble a team that best suits the person who is ill. As conditions and standards are constantly changing, consulting with professionals who are part of your team is essential.

## Standards of massage therapy practice

Professional massage therapists complete a training program that varies in length, depending on the local requirements for practice. Usually, they have to pass a board examination or national certification examination to prove that they meet the standard for safe massage therapy practice (New York State Office of the Professions 2010). They take continuing education courses and join professional massage therapy organizations to further advance their skills. Massage therapy licensing agencies and professional organizations create practice standards and codes of conduct to set expectations regarding practice and ethical conduct. While caregivers—whether family or unlicensed healthcare practitioners—are not bound by these standards, and have not completed training in massage therapy, they should know important standards and make every effort to follow the recommendations.

## Cautions and contraindications

The most important standard of care for massage therapy is knowledge about cautions and contraindications. Certain conditions require cautious use of massage to prevent harm. Modifications may include avoiding massage over certain areas, not working too deeply or eliminating certain massage therapy strokes. Contraindications are factors that render the performance of massage inadvisable given someone's state of health and current condition. If massage is contraindicated, then alternatives should be considered, such as non-moving touch, mindful presence or other ways to provide comfort.

The following lists of conditions and medications that require alternatives or adjustments to the use of massage are not exhaustive, but are part of the current standards that professional therapists follow. Though you will use light touch, will not be providing full body massage, and will proceed only with medical consent, being aware of these guidelines will help you become a more educated participant in the team. Standards change as new findings emerge, and the professionals that you work with should be familiar with the most up-to-date guidelines. It is also good to know about these guidelines should you have a professional massage for yourself.

## Contraindications

In the following circumstances, massage therapy is *contraindicated* and should not be performed.

### BLEEDING OR BLEEDING DISORDERS

People with bleeding disorders are at risk of further bleeding and bruising caused by massage. When the person is actively bleeding or when their platelets, the cells responsible for clotting the blood, are below 10,000 per microliter, the risk of injury and further damage increases, so massage should be avoided. If platelet counts are between 10,000 and 50,000 the use of very light touch, without pressure or squeezing, might be an option after getting medical clearance.

### BLOOD CLOTS

Although not common in the arms and hands, if someone has a blood clot in the area, touch or massage should be avoided completely. If there is a blood clot in the legs, you will need a physician's permission before proceeding.

### FEVER

A fever is indicative of the body's efforts to fight against an infection and inflammation. Massage can increase circulation and take away from the body's effort to fight off an infection or mount an inflammatory response. Massage should be postponed until the fever has resolved.

### FRACTURES

Massage over broken bones may cause an increase of pain in addition to the risk of further injury when pressure is applied.

## INFECTION

An infection presents an immediate challenge to the body's immune system as it mounts a response to fight the infection. Increasing circulation to the skin detracts from the body's efforts to fight off infection and is not advised as a result.

## INFLAMMATION

Inflammation causes redness, swelling and heat in areas that are affected. It can be localized to one area such as the skin or a joint or can affect the whole body. Massage therapy increases redness, heat and circulation by bringing more blood to the area being massaged. This will cause further swelling and inflammation, making massage over an inflamed area inadvisable.

## LYMPHEDEMA

Swelling caused by the removal of lymph nodes or ineffective lymphatic drainage may affect the arm. Massage cannot be performed if lymphedema is present. Lymphatic drainage performed by a trained professional can treat the lymphedema and may be recommended by the person's physician.

## MASSES

Massage in areas where there are tumors, masses, varicose veins or hernias should not be performed, as the tissues in these areas are compromised.

## PAIN

People with uncontrolled pain that is not well managed should not have massage. Managing their pain is a priority and the use of massage would not be beneficial during a crisis such as this.

## SKIN LESIONS AND CONDITIONS

Massage over rashes, wounds, recent scars or surgeries, bruises, burns, blisters and other skin lesions should not be performed.

## UNCONTROLLED SYMPTOMS

Severe symptoms that are not well managed are a priority and should be managed before offering massage. Massage therapy would not be beneficial during a crisis where the symptoms of illness are bothersome. Massage in addition to standard treatment can be very effective and result in a reduced need for higher doses of medications or more frequent use of medications to alleviate symptoms.

## *Cautions*

In the following circumstances, massage therapy may be performed using *caution*, after getting medical clearance.

### BLEEDING OR BLEEDING DISORDERS

People with platelet counts of less than 50,000 but greater than 10,000 per microliter are at risk of bleeding and bruising. When platelets are low, the risk of injury and further damage increases; however, bear in mind that you are sharing a hand massage which is almost always a safe practice. Touch should be light and used with extra care. Repeated tapping or pressure should be avoided. If a person is actively bleeding or when their platelets are below 10,000, massage is contraindicated and should not be used.

### CACHEXIA

Cachexia, wasting caused by illness and inability to eat, results in weight loss and weakness. It is most often seen in people with end-stage cancer, chronic airway disease and HIV. People who have been ill and have lost significant amounts of weight may not tolerate massage very well. Using light and superficial strokes may be all that weak and debilitated people can tolerate.

### CANCER

Comforting touch in cancer care is often used to help alleviate symptoms, however cautions should be observed. Cancer that has spread to the lymphatic system may preclude the entire area of the body affected by cancer from being massaged. When a person is undergoing cancer treatment, further cautions may apply if their blood counts are low or they are at risk for bleeding or infection. Additionally, their physician may have requirements regarding the timing of your massage if the receiver is receiving chemotherapy or radiation. Oil should not be used on the skin over areas being irradiated as this will cause a burn. Check with the physician regarding cautions before you begin.

## CHRONIC DISEASES

Chronic diseases such as diabetes, asthma and HIV may result in metabolic changes that increase the person's risk of adverse effects of massage.

## HIGH BLOOD PRESSURE

When blood pressure is high, massage should be limited to light, superficial massage.

## IMMUNO-COMPROMISED

People who are immuno-compromised are susceptible to infection. Massage therapy may be offered if the massage is modified to ensure safety. Wearing gloves may be a priority and in some instances a mask is recommended too.

## MEDICAL DEVICES

Implanted medical devices will interfere with the performance of massage, especially if they are placed in areas of the body where you plan to touch. Massage is contraindicated over implanted tubes and devices since it may cause injury to the tissues in that area. Care must be taken when massaging the surrounding skin to prevent injury. Medical devices that are not implanted should be avoided completely and care must be taken not to dislodge the device.

## NERVOUS SYSTEM DISORDERS

With nervous system disorders the receiver may have increased sensitivity to touch and their perception of pain may be augmented. Nerve pain feels like a burning or radiating pain that is very difficult to alleviate. Modifications to massage may include using certain strokes that do not increase pain. When touch to the skin causes pain, this is a good indicator that massage is not the right therapy for the person.

## OSTEOPOROSIS

Osteoporosis causes brittle bones that may break easily. Applying pressure over bones where there is evidence of osteoporosis is contraindicated and massage therapy strokes should be limited to light, superficial strokes without applying any pressure on underlying bones.

## PREGNANCY

Pregnant women, especially in the first trimester, should not have deep massage and the abdominal area must be avoided. Some meridian points should be avoided, including the Large Intestine 4 point on the hand (see p.67).

## SWELLING

Swelling or edema is of concern. The nature of the swelling should be evaluated prior to doing massage. Swelling caused by injury is handled differently than swelling caused by heart disease or by lymphatic disorders. In essence, the goal of massage should not be to move the fluid from the swollen tissues or to alleviate the swelling.

## VITAL ORGAN DISEASE

Diseases affecting vital organs such as heart disease, brain disorders, lung disease or liver disease will require a cautious approach to massage therapy. Disorders affecting vital organs have a significant effect on the body that will interfere with massage. Various symptoms will affect the ability to be comfortable during massage. People with heart and lung disease may be short of breath or get short of breath easily. People with heart disease may report chest pain and have swelling in their hands, feet and lower back. People with brain disorders may have mental status changes and are prone to seizures. People with liver disease may have mental status changes, jaundice and report itchy skin as a result. You should take into account the symptoms the receiver may be experiencing and how their disease may affect them during massage.

## *Medications*

Medications may present a risk to massage therapy also. Listed below are some of the commonly used medications that may interfere with massage and result in necessary modifications.

### BLOOD THINNERS

Blood thinning medication increases the risk of bleeding. With physician permission, you may perform light massage if the risks of bleeding are low.

### PAIN MEDICATION

Pain medications decrease the perception of pain. As a result, massage should be light and superficial.

### CHEMOTHERAPY

Chemotherapy and radiation may interfere with massage. Depending on timing and the effects of chemotherapy and radiation, massage may be contraindicated. Permission to do massage must be obtained from a physician.

### SEDATIVES

Medications that are sedating or cause drowsiness also interfere with massage. If the receiver is not able to respond and provide feedback, your massage must be light and superficial. It might be more satisfying to giver and receiver if you plan the massage session for a time when sedation is not at its greatest.

## ANTIDEPRESSANTS

Antidepressants may also have a sedating effect similar to sedatives and pain medications. If so, massage should be light and superficial. When positioning the receiver, you should bear in mind that their blood pressure may be low and changes in position may cause dizziness.

## ANTI-DIABETIC MEDICATIONS

Anti-diabetic medications assist in lowering the blood glucose level. Insulin is administered in the form of a subcutaneous injection and the receiver may be monitoring their blood sugar levels frequently. To check the blood sugar, the receiver may perform finger sticks to obtain a sample of blood. Finger sticks over an extended period will make the skin on the fingers course and hard. The tips of the fingers may be sensitive as a result. You will need to be mindful of whether the receiver is a diabetic, if they test their blood sugar frequently, how they test their blood sugar, if their last blood sugar reading was within the normal range, when they took anti-diabetic medications and how the medication affects them. If their blood sugar is low, they may have changes to their mental state and become drowsy. If the blood sugar is high, you may notice that they report being thirsty and may need to urinate frequently. If any of these circumstances occur, the management of their diabetes takes precedence over hand massage and you should not share a massage without prior permission from the receiver's physician.

## ANTI-NAUSEA MEDICATION

Anti-nausea medications alleviate nausea and associated vomiting. Some work through sedating the person and will change their perceptions. Positioning for comfort is important when the receiver is nauseous, as some positions will cause rather than alleviate retching. Frequent changes in position will also increase the possibility of nausea and vomiting. If the receiver lies with their head elevated or on their side it may help to minimize nausea, and if vomiting occurs they will not aspirate. Have an emesis bowl or towels available to use if vomiting and retching interferes with the massage.

## ANTI-HYPERTENSIVE MEDICATIONS

Anti-hypertensive medications will lower the receiver's blood pressure. Massage has a relaxing effect and may also lower blood pressure. If the receiver has taken anti-hypertensive medications within two hours of massage, you should assist them when moving from a lying to a sitting position or from a sitting to a standing position. The anti-hypertensive medications may cause a significant drop in blood pressure, making the receiver dizzy or at risk of passing out if they change position too quickly.

## STEROIDS

Steroids reduce inflammation and have an immunosuppressing effect. Using good hand hygiene and infection control practice is advised. Over a long period of time, steroids will make the skin more fragile and prone to skin tears. Massage strokes should be light and conservative over fragile skin.

## DIURETICS

Diuretics increase urinary output by filtering more blood and creating more urine. These medications are used most often in people with heart disease to reduce the accumulated fluid. When taken within a few hours of massage, the receiver may need to urinate frequently. This will interfere with the flow of massage and should be taken into account when timing the massage. These medications will also decrease the blood pressure and may cause dizziness if the blood pressure is too low.

## IMMUNOSUPPRESSANTS

Immunosuppressive drugs are used with all types of transplant, auto immune disorders and when a person is receiving chemotherapy.

These medications increase susceptibility to infection. Massage should be used conservatively with the permission of the receiver's physician.

LAXATIVES

If the receiver is constipated, they may be taking laxatives. As a result, the timing of the massage is important. Laxatives will stimulate the colon and a bowel movement usually occurs within a few hours of taking them. If you are sharing massage within a few hours of the receiver taking laxatives, you can expect that the need to visit the bathroom may interrupt the massage. These medications may also cause stomach cramps which will also interfere with the receiver's comfort during the massage.

## Alternatives to massage

When precautions are followed, massage and touch can be safe and helpful even for people with serious illnesses. Part of any safety assessment involves evaluating risk, reviewing cautions and contraindications associated with the receiver's condition and current treatment, and discussion with their healthcare team. A simple, light hand massage offers the least risk for most people and most medical conditions. As with all treatment plans, safety is the highest priority and guides the types of treatments that offer benefit and minimize risk. In research studies, injuries associated with massage are very few and usually involve localized pain or discomfort, bruising or swelling in an area where pressure is applied either too deeply or for too long.

When it is impractical for any reason to use massage strokes, an alternative to consider is 'non-moving touch'. When used as part of a therapeutic session, 'touch without movement is not casual or social touch, but is skilled touch with intention' (Tappan and Benjamin 1998, p.102). This could be simply holding hands, or just placing a hand on one area of the body. Though there may be no movement, laying the hands on the body can create warmth and a calming influence, may possibly balance energy and can have a 'personal quality not easy to describe' (Kellog cited in Tappan and Benjamin 1998, p.102). For instance, one study used 'comfort touch', which consisted of simple handshaking and patting the hand, forearm and shoulder during a five-minute social and verbal interaction (Butts 2001).

Reiki is popular among the general public and is an increasingly accepted therapy in healthcare facilities, often being incorporated into the care provided by nurses and other healthcare practitioners. Reiki was developed by a Japanese Buddhist, Mikao Usui, and involves the transfer of radiant energies through the palms (International Center for Reiki Training 2011). The practitioner's hands are placed on specific parts of the body depending on the needs of the receiver. It can also be performed with the practitioner's hands off the body, transmitting energy to the radiant field around the body. It is a gently balancing approach used to reduce pain (Olson and Hanson 1997), improve quality of life (Tsang, Carlson and Olson 2007) and facilitate a deepened awareness of spiritual connection (Gallob 2003). Though it is appreciated as an adjunct to care, the significance of Reiki use needs further study to be accepted within mainstream care. A clinical review of 205 studies on Reiki concluded that evidence was insufficient to suggest it as an effective treatment (Lee, Pittler and Ernst 2008).

Therapeutic Touch is an energy-field modality developed by Dolores Krieger that is based on several ancient healing practices. Her course, 'Frontiers in Nursing', was developed in the early 1970s and has been taught at New York University's College of Nursing and around the world ever since. The intent of the practitioner is to balance the energy flow through and around the body of the receiver. This can be done with no physical touching, or by placing the hands lightly on the shoulders, arms or legs. The receiver remains clothed and the session lasts no longer than 20 minutes (Pearce 2010).

Therapeutic Touch is an important part of wholistic nursing, with research supporting its use. It has been investigated for pain relief (Coakley and Duffy 2010; Smith, Kimmel and Milz 2010), cellular healing (Jhaveri et al. 2008) and for use with people with dementia (Woods, Beck and Sinha 2009). It has also been shown with dementia to ease restlessness (Woods, Beck and Sinha 2009) and to reduce disruptive behaviors (Hawranik, Johnston and Deatrich 2008).

These specialized forms of non-moving touch are often used in hospitals by nurses or massage therapists. If you are interested in them, you might check with your facility or healthcare team to see if someone on staff is skilled in one of these modalities and can provide guidance.

# Ethics

While sharing a hand massage, ethical practice may not be at the forefront of your mind, however, the principles of ethical conduct can be useful in your interactions with the receiver. Basic ethical practices include first obtaining permission from the receiver to provide the hand massage. When obtaining consent, it is important to explain what you will be doing in a way that the receiver can understand. When consenting, the receiver is also relating that they understand what they have been told and agree with the plan.

If the receiver is unable to give verbal consent, you should look for non-verbal indicators of consent. Watch for the nod of the head or a smile or other signs of pleasure. However, if you are not a family member, consent should be obtained from the receiver's family or healthcare proxy if the receiver is cognitively impaired. If the receiver expresses discomfort or pulls their hand away, it may indicate that they are uncomfortable. You should never continue with a massage against the will of the receiver, regardless of whether they have the capacity to consent or not.

Evaluate the acceptance of your massage throughout the session. Be sure the receiver is comfortable and that you are using the depth and the pressure appropriate for the receiver. Make adjustments as needed, or stop if necessary. Reading body language is useful when the receiver is cognitively impaired or has limited ability to communicate.

Another standard of care is creating a safe environment. A very important aspect involves preventing exposure to and transmission of infection. This includes avoiding contact with vulnerable people when you are ill so infection is not transmitted. In healthcare facilities, you will be expected to follow facility guidelines regarding wearing personal protective equipment when working with residents. This may involve wearing gloves, gowns and masks when entering the rooms of patients who have communicable diseases or are immuno-compromised. Hand washing, discussed in further detail in Chapter 8 'A Hand Massage Sequence', is the single most effective activity that promotes safety and prevents the transmission of infections and should be an important part of your use of massage.

## *Boundaries*

When you share a massage with someone you enter their personal space, touching them and entering into a relationship that may be closer than is comfortable for them. Allowing someone to share a massage requires an adjustment to usual interpersonal boundaries. These boundaries include physical, emotional and cultural barriers to name a few. There are a multitude of barriers and boundaries that are present between people, some of which are obvious, some of which are unknown.

Boundaries involve both physical and psychological components. The interplay between physical proximity, perceptions, interpersonal connections, and relationships defines interpersonal boundaries. Physical boundaries include personal space, comfort zones and proximity to others. Additionally, clothing and other objects may further impact the level of comfort experienced. Psychological boundaries are a reflection of personality and the influence of others, value systems, and cultural norms and practices. Emotional boundaries define how we feel during interpersonal contact and can be governed by the interaction (Benjamin and Sohnen-Moe 2005).

Boundaries help define identity, integrity and relationships, and differ vastly from one person to the next. Assessing the boundaries and levels of comfort between you and the receiver is an important aspect of massage. One way to think about boundaries is to assess your own: What boundaries do you have? Are you shy? Do you maintain eye contact when talking to someone? Do some people stand too close to you or touch you when you are not open to touch? Then you can consider the receiver's perceptions: What boundaries are evident with the person with whom you will share a massage? Are they more comfortable with a male or a female giver? Does their cultural background influence the relationship? Does their age make a difference to the way they perceive your touch?

If you are unsure about someone's boundary needs, you can begin conservatively and gradually, assessing the receiver's response as you go.

## Transference

Transference occurs when the giver or receiver have perceptions, thoughts and feelings that are not based on reality or information that is true, but on a projection they are making. For example, the giver may assume that people with cancer have pain all the time and as a result, feel upset about their suffering. This is a general assumption made on the part of the giver that may not be true for the receiver. This is a transferential experience based on information unrelated to the current massage therapy relationship.

Similarly, the receiver may have a transferential experience related to the massage and/or the giver. A common example of this would be the receiver's perception that massage is a sexual experience.

In circumstances where transference is evident, the giver is advised to be mindful of their thoughts and assumptions about the receiver and to maintain appropriate boundaries and behavior. If transference is evident on the part of the receiver, it may be important to manage their expectations about the massage therapy experience by clarifying your intention to provide comfort.

## WHEN SHARING TOUCH:
## LEARN TO TRUST YOURSELF

Ms. M. went to the emergency room because she was having trouble breathing. The doctors quickly diagnosed pneumonia. Her age of 87, plus a history of heart failure, made this a precarious situation for her. After talking to the family, the do not resuscitate (DNR) order was rescinded to allow a breathing tube to be inserted temporarily, to see if Ms. M. would improve when the pneumonia was treated. She was admitted to the intensive care unit.

Her two daughters were by her side on a daily basis. Due to the tube, Ms. M. was sedated to ensure her comfort. She had intravenous medication lines in her neck, arm and leg. The doctors identified a highly contagious virus as the possible cause, so when visiting their mother the daughters had to wear gloves, a mask and a gown.

One of the daughters, Sarah, had learned the comforting touch sequence. But at this time she had no desire to use it, despite the value she felt it could have. Sarah herself was feeling weak, having just had the flu. In addition, all of the tubes concerned her, and she was upset that this time no amount of medical care would rescue her mom, who had made surprising recoveries in the past.

Sarah accepted the situation and did not force the issue. Massage just didn't feel right to her. So she simply placed her hands on her mother's arm and hand that had no medical lines inserted. She and her sister spoke to their mother, even though she was unconscious, while they visited her.

One afternoon, after a week of hospitalization, Sarah was alone in the room with her mother. There was no clarity about what might happen with her mother, only educated speculation; the medical team felt Ms. M. was doing well enough to remove the breathing tube, but was not sure which day they would attempt it. Sarah had to leave the next day to go back home and didn't know when she could return. She realized that this might be the last time she would have with her mother.

As she held her mother's hand in hers, Sarah closed her eyes and tried some breathing to relax. After a few conscious breaths she had a quick image of her mother, a photo of her when she was about 13. Sarah decided to 'meet' her mom as a teenager, and imagined asking, 'Were you a rebellious kid like me?' She imagined her mother replying, 'No, I think I was more scared than rebellious.' Sarah, who had given her parents a hard time during her teen years, reflected back and replied, 'I guess I was pretty scared too.'

Then she continued the waking dream, imaging her mother growing up, becoming a young mother, her years of working nights to help support the family. It was a long perspective she had never had before, a more complete reality of all they had shared through the years. This was a new sense of relationship that would remain with Sarah even after her mother died, which she did, three weeks later. Though not conscious of it at the time, Sarah's decision not to focus on the body had provided a way for her to connect to essence.

## THE INNER PRACTICE:
## BREATHING IN HARMONY

The imagination is a great access to the inner world. Psychologist Catherine Shainberg, director of the School of Images in New York City, teaches that access to the imagination—its images, sounds and smells—takes place through an open, relaxed watching. Imagination is differentiated from illusions, projections and fantasies through a body-centered awareness that allows the practitioner to distinguish habitual surface reactions from true intuitive feelings. 'In thus securing our imagination to the movements of the body, we clear our inner screen to reflect the wisdom that is waiting to shine through' (Shainberg 2005, p.15).

This is an exercise Dr. Shainberg teaches in her classes. The exercise is neither difficult nor time consuming. It takes just a few moments of focusing. Read the exercise. Then sit in a comfortable position with your feet on the floor and hands resting on your thighs. If you are comfortable, close your eyes.

1. Take a breath in, mindfully and fully. You imagine, as you continue breathing in and out, that you are breathing in harmony with all the different parts of yourself becoming one.

   ∘ See, sense and feel that you are breathing in harmony with everyone in the room.

   ∘ See, sense and feel that you are breathing in harmony with all those you love.

   ∘ See, sense and feel that you are breathing in harmony with all those you know.

- ° See, sense and feel that you are breathing in harmony with all people in the world.

2. Breathe out, with a slow and mindful exhalation.

   - ° You imagine, as you continue breathing in and out, that you are breathing in harmony with the animals you love.

   - ° See, sense and feel that you are breathing in harmony with all animal life.

3. Breathe out, with a slow and mindful exhalation.

   - ° You imagine, as you continue breathing in and out, that you are breathing in harmony with all of the plants in your house.

   - ° See, sense and feel that you are breathing in harmony with all plant life.

4. See, sense and feel that you are breathing in harmony with all of Nature.

5. Observe what you feel and sense in your body. Breathe out mindfully and open your eyes.

(Used with permission of Catherine Shainberg.)

# Chapter 7

# Elements of
# a Session

Creative freedom, ironically, is born of discipline. Popular songs, for instance, which seem so free spirited, have every 'yeah, yeah, yeah' planned out in the sheet music. The framework allows for complexity to be contained into a coherent message.

Before you share a massage, take some time to think it through to enhance your vision of what and how you want to communicate. By focusing ahead of time—giving some thought to your intentions, supplies needed, comfort for the receiver and yourself—you will create the safety and predictability that support the flow of heartfelt feelings.

## What do you want to communicate?

What kind of 'spirit' do you want to bring to the time you will spend sharing touch? If your intent is to share a relaxing massage, you will prepare with an inner practice that focuses on calming, and as an external preparation you might consider dimming the lights, playing soft, slow music and moving quietly around the room. You might bring battery-operated candles in to create a soft glow in the room. You could close the door to keep out distracting sounds and smells.

If you plan an engaging, light-hearted massage experience, you may decide to be more verbal, engage the receiver in conversation if possible, be more communicative, keep the lights on in the room and avoid using music since it might interfere with the conversation. You can choose, or change, depending on what is appropriate for the receiver.

Sometimes the receiver will want to chat more, at least in the beginning. It is best to follow their lead. Whichever intention you choose, maintain eye contact, watch for the receiver's responses and proceed slowly and gently.

## Rhythm of the session

The timing of the massage during the day is a factor worth considering. Is it better to offer massage first thing in the morning, or after the receiver has had breakfast and washed up for the day? Are there times during the day when they are bored or seem to be uncomfortable and therefore might benefit from massage at those times? Would they be more receptive when they are out of bed and sitting in a chair? Or would a 20-minute massage in the early evening help them to sleep better during the night?

You might wonder how long you should spend sharing the hand massage. This will vary, again, depending on the receiver, the time of day and what is happening in the environment. The sequence provides a framework for 30 minutes of shared activity as an ideal. In real life, you may start out with only a few minutes. If the receiver is agitated and prefers to walk, for instance, a minute may be all you can manage. Or, the receiver may have contractures, and you are limited in the kinds of stroke you can perform. Maybe you feel you just don't have the time. Research on hand massage for a variety of populations has found benefits when shared for as little as five minutes total (Butts 2001), but most commonly it was used for about 10–20 minutes (Harris and Richards 2010).

## Gathering supplies

Depending on where the receiver will be situated for the massage, either in bed or sitting in a chair, there are a number of supplies that will help to make the massage as comfortable as possible. Pillows or a soft cushion may be helpful to bolster the arms. Pillows are usually readily available, whether the receiver is at home or in a facility. As mentioned above, depending on the nature of the session you plan, you might also bring into the room a CD player or battery-powered candles.

No lotion is required for the hand massage described. However, you may want to use a lotion as another element than can be soothing. People who are ill may be sensitive to lotions, creams and smells. Err on the side of caution to begin with and choose a basic unscented lotion or oil, should you decide to use one. If the receiver is in a facility, you may be restricted to an approved lotion that the facility can provide. Check with the care team before using any lotion.

Using gloves during the massage may be required if the person who is ill is immuno-compromised, has a communicable illness, or their condition increases your risk of contact with body fluids. The healthcare team will advise you whether gloves are needed based on the receiver's medical condition, in addition to using your better judgment in deciding whether gloves are needed.

Performing massage while wearing gloves is much different than performing massage without gloves. Gloves are a barrier to feeling and connecting with the skin, and they may not move easily over the skin unless you use lotion or oil. If you need to wear gloves, practice the protocol ahead of time while wearing the gloves so that you become proficient in doing massage while wearing them.

## The goals of care

We all have hopes and expectations for our lives and prioritize what is important to us. Our personal values and beliefs guide us in making decisions, including health care decisions that are right for us. Whenever illness or deteriorating health becomes a factor in our lives, our hopes and priorities change to include managing the illness and the challenges it presents in our daily lives. When these choices are shared with the healthcare team, they become part of the goals of care (Robert H. Lurie Comprehensive Cancer Center of Northwestern University 2004). 'Goals of care' is a defined clinical term based on what the receiver wants. Anyone providing massage should follow goals of care, which means following the wishes of the receiver.

For instance, caregivers who are anxious about ways to help the person who is ill often turn to food as a way to express their love and will cook the ill person's favorite meals. This may become a contentious activity, since the sick person may not have an appetite or the ability to eat the meal. A good solution to alleviating caregiver distress is to channel their urge to cook into an urge to touch. Caregivers who learn the massage protocol learn a valuable tool that enables them to alleviate their distress about providing something helpful while at the same time honoring the current needs and wants of the receiver.

Identifying the goals of massage helps to focus your intention on providing a massage experience that meets the receiver's needs. Your primary intention is to comfort and connect. You do not need to feel that you have to 'get results', but you can be mindful of how massage helps to alleviate or reduce some symptoms they may be experiencing, how the strokes bring about relaxation, how an agitated mind can be coaxed into focusing on touch, or how your presence can create a shared feeling of well-being. The goals of care may also center around spending time together, helping the person who is ill not feel like a burden and promoting the enjoyment of visitors.

# The plan of care

Once you have determined the goals of care—your hopes for massage and your intention in sharing massage—these goals guide the plan of care. The plan of care is essentially how you will achieve the goals, the steps you use and your approach to sharing massage that you think will bring about the desired results.

Massage therapy is more often than not a welcome addition to the medical plan of care and a valuable palliative treatment. Palliative care is one aspect of health care that focuses on alleviating pain and symptoms associated with disease. It supports decision making that is in line with personal values and improves quality of life. It brings a meaningful, effective therapy into a person's life that they can look forward to and enjoy while also reaping physical, energetic and spiritual benefits.

A friend or family member can provide a unique addition to the care plan when they offer focused touch that helps to palliate the receiver's symptoms. They may be able to offer it more frequently and for a greater length of time than any member of the medical team could. Working collaboratively with the medical team will help you formulate your therapeutic approach and the intent of your hand massage as part of the bigger picture in improving the receiver's quality of life. Perhaps you can encourage other caregivers or family members to learn the massage protocol so they can also offer support and connection through touch.

## The importance of recognizing individual needs

In a wholistic approach to health care there is no one answer. The individual's needs are the center of concern. Those needs will vary and keep changing. The receiver's medical history or an acute health-related situation may change how you perform the massage and may require you to be cautious or to decide to forgo massage.

Certain illnesses and their treatment, diseases affecting the hands, and the medical plan of care should be considered before you consider massage. If you are sharing massage in a facility, you should consult with the facility care team about any new situations that affect the receiver. For instance, if the receiver has a fever or has been bothered by recent symptoms that are likely to interfere with the massage, it might not be appropriate.

Always consult with the receiver's physician or healthcare team before performing massage so you can get their permission and guidance about what will best suit the receiver given his or her current medical condition. While the hands are among the safest places in the body to touch when the receiver is frail or ill, the giver must still be mindful about ensuring that the benefits of massage outweigh the risks and that the receiver will be able to tolerate massage. Refer to Chapter 6 'Before You Begin' for details on cautions and contraindications that should be observed.

Once you have medical consent, you will assess the receiver's arms and hands before doing massage. Pay attention to the quality of their skin, the way they position their arms, and barriers or challenges to performing the sequence of steps described in Chapter 8. Check for dryness of the skin, rashes, swelling, bumps, bruises, lesions or wounds that may interfere with the massage. Swelling in the joints and hands, pain in the hands, redness, or heat to touch may preclude you from offering massage, since these are signs and symptoms indicative of inflammation. If you see any of these visible signs, speak to the physician before you proceed.

Modifications to the hand massage protocol will also be needed if the receiver has contractures in their arms and hands. You should not reposition their arms, but should limit your massage strokes to the areas you can touch easily.

Sometimes the receiver may have tubes and devices that are used in the treatment of their illness. Tubes and devices located in the arms, or devices in other areas of the body that interfere with access to the arms and hands, will also require changes in what you do. Modifications you might need to make based on various conditions are discussed in greater detail in Chapter 11 'Adapting for Different Needs'.

# Preparing yourself
## Contraindications and cautions for the giver
Caregivers who provide massage should consider their own health, state of mind and ability as well. If you have any of the contraindications or cautions that are mentioned in Chapter 6 'Before You Begin', consult your physician, as illnesses and medications will affect your ability to share touch. If you have recently had a big meal or have been drinking alcohol you should wait until you are no longer under the influence before offering massage.

## *Hand hygiene*

Washing your hands prior to offering massage is an essential practice to reduce the transmission of infection and other micro-organisms from one person to another. In healthcare facilities, the risks of transmission are much higher than in the home, as there are a number of people in close proximity to each other that are being cared for by healthcare practitioners who move from one person to another. Additionally, people who are ill are at higher risk of contracting an infection purely because their immune system is compromised by their illness or treatment. Careful hand washing is a must before and after your massage. As you wash your hands, whether at home or in a healthcare facility, you can use those moments to also center yourself and focus your mind. See 'When sharing touch: Wash your hands first' in Chapter 8 for hand-washing guidelines from the Center for Disease Control and Prevention (2010) and the World Health Organization (2009a, b).

## *Healthy hands*

Massage therapists take good care of their hands. They follow recommendations about hand hygiene before and after massage and groom their hands and nails consistently. Fingernails should be kept short and should not extend beyond the tips of the fingers. This minimizes the risk of injury to the receiver when sharing massage. The area under the fingernails is a common area that harbors dirt, fungus and bacteria. A healthy practice includes frequent cleaning with soap, water and a nail brush. Artificial nails or wraps increase the presence of bacteria on the fingernails and can pose the risk of infection. Similarly, nail polish can also harbor bacteria. Use your discretion about wearing artificial nails or nail polish, but if you do so be sure to wash your hands and fingernails thoroughly.

Rings and bracelets can increase the risk of injury and infection. When sharing massage, the giver should be mindful to remove jewelry before washing hands and beginning the massage sequence. If you are unable to remove the jewelry, pay particular attention to washing the jewelry with a nail brush in addition to washing your hands. When sharing massage, ensure the jewelry does not scrape or tear the receiver's skin. Massage may not be appropriate if the jewelry you are wearing cannot be removed or has surfaces that can cause injury.

## Enter mindfully

Once you have consulted with the healthcare team, prepared the supplies you will need, and washed your hands, you are ready to enter the room. When walking into the room, you enter the person's personal space. For someone in a facility, their bed and night table may be the only personal space they have left. The etiquette of entering the room, whether it is in their home or in a facility, is to be respectful of this space and obtain permission to enter.

You may do this by knocking on the door first and standing in the doorway until they look in your direction and acknowledge your presence. You may need to call to them, say their name and raise your voice a little, so you can get their attention. Once their attention is on you, ask if you may enter and wait for their response.

As you approach the receiver, you already begin to touch them with your presence. A person's individual personal safety zone may expand or shrink depending on their situation. Having someone in close physical proximity may cause stress, or it may be perceived as tolerable or even comforting (Vortherms 1991). It is not recommended to enter the room freely, speak loudly or make a lot of noise that will startle the person.

If the person is sleeping and your knocking and calling from the doorway does not arouse them, you should consider the individual situation. If they are sleeping frequently, you might enter the room and touch them gently to awaken them. On the other hand, you may not want to wake them if they are often agitated or have trouble sleeping; in that case you may want to return when they are awake.

When entering the room, you will want to take in the big picture, evaluating the overall impression you get. Where is the person? Are they in bed or sitting in a chair? How do they look? Do they seem happy, sad, content, uncomfortable, peaceful, depressed, anxious, in pain or sedated? How are they positioned? Are they sitting comfortably, or are they sliding down in the chair? Do they need pillows and bolsters to support them? Are they able to maintain their position independently? Are they clean and well groomed? These initial impressions influence what steps you might take in making the receiver comfortable, as well as how you will share a massage with them.

## Creating the right conditions
### *Greeting the receiver*

As you enter, if the person is verbal, you might ask how they are feeling, how their day has been so far, if they are experiencing any pain, discomfort or other symptoms, and if they have taken any recent medications. Getting a clear picture about how the receiver is feeling is most helpful. Of interest are medications for the management of pain that may alter their sensation during the massage. Medications to help alleviate anxiety may affect their wakefulness and ability to provide feedback during the massage.

As you greet the receiver, their response will give you insight into their mood, whether or not they are able to communicate with you, and how they might be feeling. Do they look you in the eye? Do they verbalize a greeting in return? Do they respond in a manner that seems confused? Is their face expressive? Do they smile when they greet you? Does the intonation and strength of their voice give you any information about their mood? Are their eyes bright and engaged or are they empty and sad?

Awareness of your own feelings and thoughts about the person as you greet them is also helpful. Do you feel their warmth and feel welcome in their space? Do you feel sad because they look sad? Does the medical equipment around them make you feel nervous and scared? While your perceptions and thoughts about the person's mood may not be completely accurate, they are, however, a barometer of your internal processing of the situation, which you may need to manage in order to get to a centered state of mind before sharing massage.

## *Preparing the receiver for massage*

You will want to explain to the receiver that you would like to provide massage for them and obtain their permission to proceed. Preparing the receiver involves explaining the hand massage protocol to them using language and terminology they can understand. If the receiver has cognitive barriers and has a limited ability to understand, you will need to explain slowly and evaluate how they perceive your explanation.

Approach the receiver in a friendly way, greeting them by name and then asking permission to proceed. For instance: 'Harriet, would it be all right if I held your hand for a while? I'd like to provide some comforting touch for you.' You can describe what you will do, that you'll be touching her arm and hand, and that you intend to be gentle. Provide the opportunity for the receiver to ask questions and answer her to the best of your ability.

Explaining the protocol can be helpful to receivers who are cautious about touch and who need to know the steps in the process before consenting. Explaining the steps to them will help to alleviate any anxiety or fear that they may have about being touched. By explaining the steps to the receiver, and having them agree with the plan, you are obtaining informed consent. This means that they understand what you have explained and are allowing you to proceed with the massage. Even if the person may seem to not hear, see or acknowledge you, assume that on some level they sense what is happening. If you are not a family member and the receiver is non-verbal or is in a comatose state, you will need to seek consent from a family member or medical professional in charge of the care plan before you proceed.

## *Make the receiver comfortable*

Having come to a verbal agreement and a level of understanding about how the massage will progress, you consider the comfort of the receiver during the massage. Ensuring that the receiver remains comfortable throughout the course of the massage is a priority. You can begin by asking the receiver how they are feeling, if there is anything bothering them, or anything that should be addressed before you start the massage. Find out whether they are having a hard time with symptoms and need treatment. If so, and you are not involved with making decisions about their treatment, you should contact the decision makers or caregivers responsible for their care before doing the massage.

The receiver may want to use the bathroom or even wash up before you begin. Perhaps they are thirsty and a sip of water is better now rather than interrupting the massage to have a drink later. They may want you to close the door, turn off the light, turn off the television, unplug the phone or even place a 'Do Not Disturb' sign on the door, to help minimize interruptions during the course of the massage.

In interacting with them, you will be further assessing their level of understanding of massage and their ability to make their needs known. You will also see whether they have a strong sense about what they want from the massage and whether they are able to direct their care. If you find that your intentions are different from the receiver's, bear in mind that the massage is tailored for them and that the best situation when sharing massage is the sharing of common goals.

You can provide the hand massage while the person is sitting in a chair, wheelchair, or is in bed. Check that the arm and hand are in a natural position. If the receiver is able to move freely, you should ask them to position themselves in a manner that is most comfortable for them. While you do the massage, make sure the receiver's forearm and hand rests on something, either on their lap, on the bed, or on the arm of the chair. Bolsters and pillows can be used to support the arm and hand and facilitate relaxation. Something as simple as having the receiver's arm in a position of comfort can make all the difference in their enjoyment of the massage experience.

It is common for the receiver to try to assist you in the massage by holding the arm up in the air. Notice if this is happening. If it is, encourage the receiver to place their arm back down, or provide support for it with one of your hands. You might even need to tell them not to help you by lifting their arm.

The room temperature may influence the receiver's comfort. If it is cold, maintain warmth for the receiver by exposing only the area on the arms and hands that you are working on. If the temperature is too hot, you may not need a blanket or cover, but you should offer its use and check in with the receiver periodically about how the temperature feels. If at any time you observe goose bumps on the receiver's arms, it may occur as a result of the temperature being too cold, but can also occur as a reaction to the massage.

If the receiver is not able to communicate with you verbally, perhaps because they are cognitively impaired or are comatose, you have to observe their responses carefully to be sure they are enjoying what you are doing. Touch is not for everyone. The intended receiver might not want massage at the moment, or at all, and that is completely acceptable. Some signs of displeasure would be words like 'no', as well as gestures of pulling away, a grimace, a moan, a clenched mouth, a clenched fist, or other expressions of discomfort. This would require you to stop and consider an alternative to touch. Or, you could try again at a different time.

## *Make yourself comfortable*

While the receiver's comfort is your priority, you should also be positioned comfortably so you can concentrate on communicating a relaxed feeling as you provide the massage. Once you have assisted the receiver into a comfortable position you can then concentrate on positioning yourself comfortably as well.

You can best perform the hand massage protocol from a seated position. You will need to use a hard chair or stool to seat yourself close to the side of the bed or chair. Hospital beds, used most frequently in facilities, may be raised or lowered to a level that works for you. The receiver's arm and hand should be close enough to you to reach comfortably.

Sitting on the bed is not advised, as this position may overstep the receiver's personal space, may not be a good idea if the receiver is very ill and has a number of medical devices and tubes, is incontinent, has wounds that produce exudate, or if the facility does not permit anyone other than the resident to sit on the bed.

ELEMENTS OF A SESSION

If you are unable to sit, try to perform the massage while standing without bending over. This will prevent muscle fatigue and back pain throughout the session. Moving your body as one unit will also spread the burden of muscle use and fatigue when standing. You can lean slightly against the receiver's bed or chair as a support.

Monitor your own comfort throughout the massage, and do not overextend yourself. Just as you should stop when the receiver expresses discomfort, you should take a break when you need to as well. It is better to do a few minutes when you are in a good place and have time, than to force any situation. Heed the experience of one caregiver, who was sharing the hand massage with a nursing home resident who was relaxing into a contented state until the caregiver realized she had to attend to something else and sped up at the end. The receiver got startled, pulled her hand away and started yelling.

# After the session
## *Leaving the room*
At the end of the massage, make sure the receiver is safe and comfortable before you leave. If the receiver is in bed and you lowered the side rails to facilitate the massage, you will need to return the railings to their original position. This prevents the receiver from falling out of bed or climbing out of bed; safety is something you should be vigilant about. You will also need to adjust the bed back to its original position if you raised or lowered it. Gather up any of the supplies you used, dispose of gloves or gowns properly if they were needed. Make sure everything that the receiver needs has been put back within reach, including their call bell if they are in a facility.

## *Contemplating the meaning of your massage*
How might you evaluate the effects of your touch? You can use your evaluation of the receiver before you began your massage to compare with an assessment you make at the end of the session, or over the course of several sessions. A study in Australia that had

111

caregivers contribute to the design, implementation and evaluation of a hand treatment for people with dementia compared some of the following behaviors before and after the massage:

- smiling

- wandering

- restlessness

- excessive daytime sleeping

- interest in activities

- initiation of conversation

- initiation of touch

- prompted memories.

Caregivers in the group recorded changes in notebooks, which became a valuable part of the research. Analysis of the data collected showed that the treatment helped caregivers to become calmer, to develop a greater sense of control over their situation and to reflect on negative attitudes. All found the treatment soothing and pleasant to use (Kilstoff and Chenoweth 1998).

After providing comforting touch, you could observe some of the behaviours listed above, as well as changes in the receiver's breathing pattern, facial expression or muscle tension. Sometimes changes are subtle, and easy to miss. But sometimes we need to be careful that we are not just looking for what we want to see. For instance, during one supervised session a daughter providing hand massage for her mother was so intent on eliciting a verbal response from her mother, that she completely missed the fact that her mother's arms, which had been positioned tightly against her chest, had relaxed down to her sides.

You might observe energetic changes, such as the warmth of the fingertips, the light in the eyes, if there is a change in tone in the voice. Is there a change in the shared field of the room? Do others feel it too?

You might evaluate yourself before and after a massage. How does your breathing change, your muscle tension, your thought process? Did you enjoy the time; was it soothing? Do you feel closer to the receiver? Did you have a brief respite from the usual worries that you have? The pleasures of touch should provide a way to relax and to connect to one another. Creating a structured approach from beginning to end will, ironically, give you the freedom to tap into a creative way of sharing life's most intimate moments.

## When sharing touch: A receiver's perspective

Janel was diagnosed with pancreatic cancer and after a course of chemotherapy she underwent major surgery followed by complications that kept her in hospital for over a month. As part of the integrative service offered by her hospital, she was visited by a massage therapist.

'In the midst of being half out of my mind because of the pain and the drugs and everything else, I had a massage therapist show up who massaged my feet and ankles for about 20–30 minutes, using very gentle touch,' Janel recalled. The massage therapist came several times during Janel's lengthy stay in the hospital. This became an island of respite for her, and something she began to look forward to. The massage was very light and the therapist wore surgical gloves, which were appropriate because of Janel's condition.

'The massage was a way to get me out of my head and into my body,' said Janel. 'That was the best thing anyone could do for me at that point. Holding the feet or the hands is so helpful because they are such a tangible way to ground a person in the body. And I didn't need anyone to speak much, because words would have kept me in my head.'

A friend who was a frequent visitor also used touch. Though she wasn't a licensed massage therapist, she had taken an introductory class for massage for personal use. Janel remembered fondly, 'She would come in and say to me, "How many feet do you have today?" or, "How many hands?" And if I said four hands she would rub one hand, then the other, and then start over again until she massaged my hands four times. She would spend a half hour that way. It was a lifesaver. The repetition was great, because she would do it until *I* was done, not until *she* was done.'

That friend was one of the few people who made Janel feel she could just be a receiver. 'There were some friends, even though I love them, who made me feel exhausted after their visit,' she said. 'The people I welcomed back were the ones who didn't need my energy to entertain them.'

The whole experience, in fact, made her realize that receiving care could be meaningful. 'I was lying there in complete misery and had a realization. There are two types of people in a hospital, those giving care and those receiving care. Caregivers can't give it unless there are people who want to receive it. I realized I had a purpose in lying there helplessly and it was to receive care. With that thought, I became an active receiver, rather than a passive one.'

When both people are present, not holding back and letting themselves be wholly in the moment, that is when the deep, transformative work happens. And there is nothing better, when you give wholeheartedly, than to be met with a wholehearted receiver.

Chapter 8

# A Hand Massage Sequence

The following steps guide you through a comforting touch session that can take up to 15 minutes for each hand, or about 20–30 minutes if you can do both hands. The touch varies, starting with gentle stroking, massaging, holding points and then stroking again. The sequence described is for an ideal situation, but it is intended to be a flexible guideline. While it provides a focus, it can be freely adapted as necessary for individual needs.

## Preparation

Chapters 6 and 7 explain in detail important ways to prepare for a hand massage session. To summarize:

- Consult with the healthcare team regarding any cautions or contraindications that may apply to your situation. Follow their recommendations.

- Remember your intention is to comfort and communicate. Take a few moments to center yourself before you begin. Proceed gently and 'give as a receiver', which means you are not only doing the strokes, but you are also receptive to sensation—such as warmth or coolness, softness or tension—that are part of the hands you are touching. Think of your touch as a process of wordless communication, with information flowing both ways.

- Consider the elements of a session, such as things to get organized and how you will greet the receiver. This includes being sure to enter the room mindfully and explaining what you are going to do, even if you think the receiver will not comprehend what you say. Remember that with focused touch you will be addressing physical, energetic and spiritual dimensions, so awareness is always present, even if it is not apparent. Proceed if the receiver is receptive.

- Carefully wash your hands and remove jewelry.

You can begin on either the right or left side of the receiver. Sit down on the side that you will be working on. Position yourself alongside the receiver so that you face them and can easily reach both their shoulder and their hand easily. Their arm should be relaxed, resting on their lap, the bed, or the arm of a chair. Assess the condition of the receiver's arms and hands and be aware of areas to avoid. You can use a pillow to prop the lower arm and hand for greater comfort, if necessary. Pay attention to your own comfort as well, and move around as necessary so your body can be relaxed while you work.

# The hand massage

## 1. Start with a feathery stroke that says hello

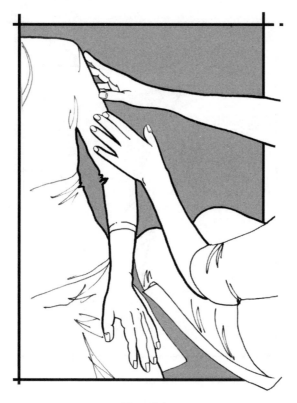

*Figure 7.1*

Use very light touch, using your fingertips like feathers as you stroke the arm from the shoulder down to the hand as a way to initiate your touch conversation. This kind of light touch stimulates the part of the nervous system that allows us to be oriented in space by activating receptors in the muscles, ligaments and bones called *proprioceptors*. A gentle touch to the arm or shoulder has been shown to be well accepted by residents in a nursing home, who perceive it as a gesture of comfort and care (Moore and Gilbert 1995).

## 2. Create some warmth by circular rubbing around the big joints

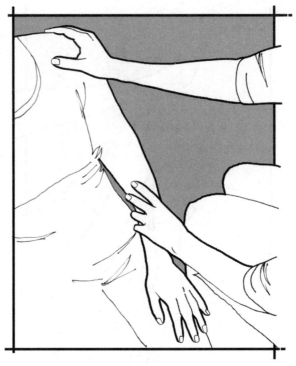

*Figure 7.2*

Rubbing the joints helps the energy flow through them more freely. Begin with the largest joint, the shoulder. The receiver's arm should be resting comfortably, in whatever position makes sense for them. The receiver's arm and hand may be on the bed or be supported by the armrest of a chair or wheelchair. The receiver should not have to hold their arm up.

Use your hand with the palm facing the shoulder (for instance, if you are sitting on the receiver's left side, use your right hand) to cup the shoulder and make slow, gentle circles over it. You can place your other hand on the arm somewhere to provide a feeling of connection and support.

Next, cup the elbow with the same hand you used for the shoulder and make slow, circular gestures around it. This can be performed over clothing if the receiver is wearing long sleeves.

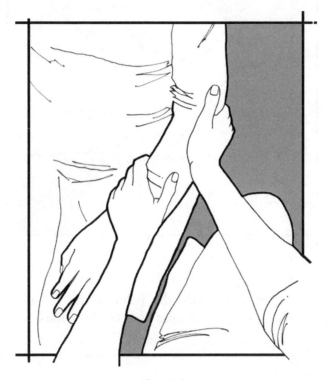

*Figure 7.3*

Finally, make circular movements over the top of the wrist. Your other hand might support the hand from underneath, or if the receiver's arm is resting on something you can place your fingers over their fingers (see Figure 7.4).

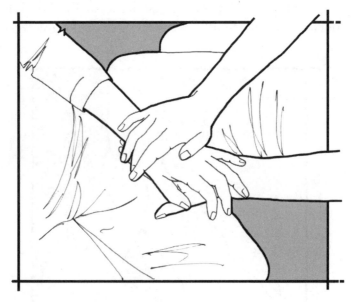

*Figure 7.4*

**3. Support the hand with the palm facing down and do small warming circular strokes over the knuckles**

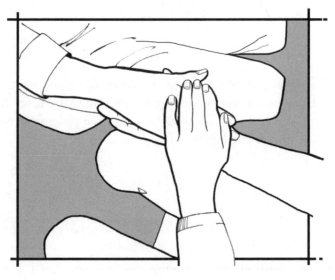

*Figure 7.5*

Let your hand rest across the knuckles and use a slow, circular motion to warm the area slightly. No need to use pressure. Be careful over knuckles, especially if they are arthritic, swollen or deformed. Don't try to straighten fingers out or place the fingers in any position.

*Reminder:* Give as a receiver. What do you feel as you stroke over the fingers? Are there differences in temperature from one finger to another? Just observe differences without trying to 'do' anything about them.

## 4. Use gliding strokes over the top of the hand

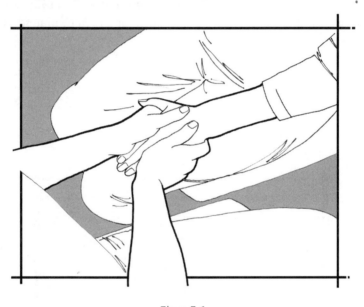

*Figure 7.6*

The basic stroke of massage that initiates the relaxation response is a gliding stroke (effleurage) along or across the muscles. Since the hand is a small area, you can use your thumbs to do the stroking to the back of the hand.

First, take a look at the back of the hand for areas where there may be rashes, lesions or sores, which you will avoid. For most people, the back of the hand does not have much flesh and the elderly will also have large veins or vein threads in this area. So apply no pressure, just use soothing, gliding strokes from the center of the hand out to the sides, as if you were applying lotion to the skin.

Start at the upper hand (near the wrist). Supporting the hand with your fingers, use your thumbs to stroke gently from the center out to the sides of the hand. When moving your thumbs, move your entire hand rather than just your thumbs. This will prevent fatigue in your thumbs. Do a few strokes and then move your thumbs to the middle of the hand to repeat the gliding strokes, and finish at the lower end of the hand just above the finger webs. There is no set rule about how many times to do this, but as a starting point use at least three strokes across each area, for a total of nine strokes across the hand.

*Reminder:* Get feedback from the receiver or observe them to assess their comfort with what you are doing. You can skip any part of the sequence that is not feasible to do.

**5. Use gliding strokes across the palm**

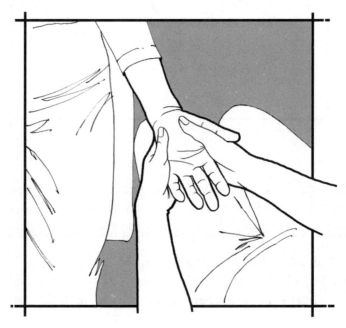

*Figure 7.7*

If possible, slowly turn the receiver's hand, thumb upwards, so the palm faces up. Put your thumbs together in the center of the palm, and then glide out from the center toward the sides of the hand. Apply gliding strokes across each section of the palm. There is usually a bit more flesh in the palm, so the gliding strokes may feel more connected.

Start at the top (just below the wrist). As you come across the palm, go into the 'pad' of the palm at the base of the thumb. After a few strokes across the top of the palm, go to the center, and then to the bottom of the palm, over the pads that lead to the fingers.

## 6. Stroke down the fingers

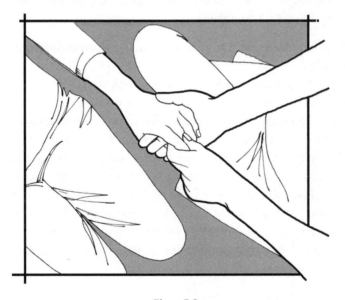

*Figure 7.8*

As you move toward the fingers, your gestures become more focused. You can stroke the fingers with either the palm up or down. The receiver's ability to turn the palm over, or not, is one consideration. Another way to choose: does the person need to 'open up to the world'? Then stroke the fingers with the palm up. If the person seems scattered and distracted, and would benefit from focusing inward, then choose to stroke the fingers with the palm down.

Supporting the hand, gently stroke each finger from knuckle to fingertip. You can do this in a variety of ways, depending on what feels good to you. You can:

- glide down the finger making a long, sweeping stroke from top to tip

- make small circles along the sides of the fingers as you glide down

- or do intermittent pressure as you go down the finger, a kind of 'walking'.

Do each finger one at a time. Do not squeeze the finger, as that will most likely elicit a complaint.

### 7. Explore the meridian points near the thumb, wrist, pinky and palm

You can choose one or more points, but you will have the best effect if you can maintain contact with a point for at least one to three minutes. You may want to choose different points depending on the moment—either what feels 'right' or what is needed.

You may find yourself drawn to one point in particular all the time, or at a certain time. Learning to follow your intuition is part of the pleasurable process of giving through touch. See the box 'The inner practice' at the end of this chapter for guidance on the quality of touch you can use when working with energy.

Chapter 5 has more detail about the point locations and benefits. In brief, they are:

- Large Intestine 4 (near the thumb) for digestion, elimination or pain. *Note:* This point cannot be used when someone is pregnant.

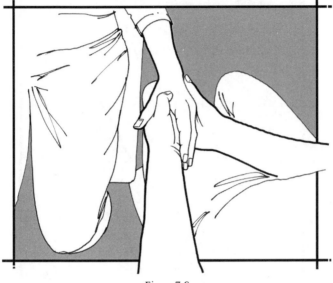

*Figure 7.9*

- Pericardium 6 (near the inner wrist) for nausea.

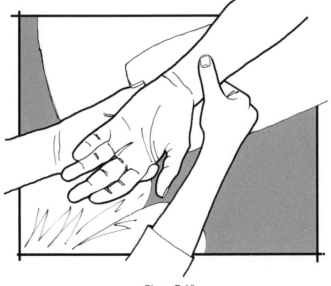

*Figure 7.10*

- Pericardium 8 (on the palm) for fatigue or anxiety.

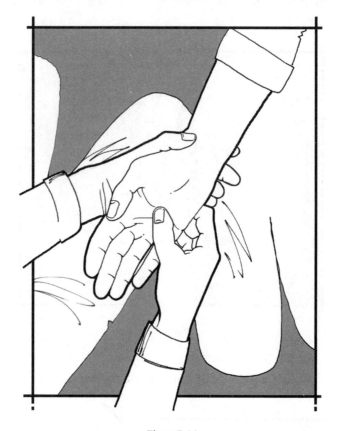

*Figure 7.11*

- Small Intestine 3 (near the pinky) for the neck and back.

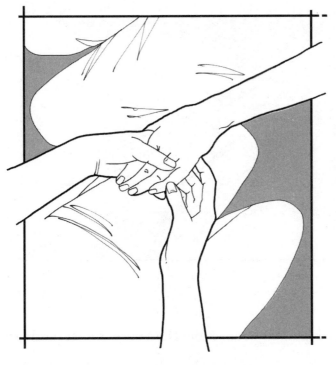

*Figure 7.12*

- Triple Warmer 4 (at the wrist) for relaxing muscles and increasing energy.

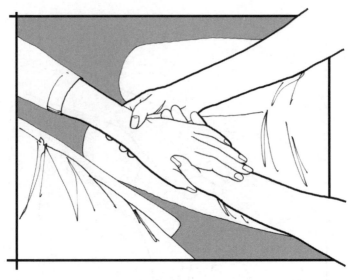

*Figure 7.13*

## 8. Maintain the connection: Hold the points at the fingertips

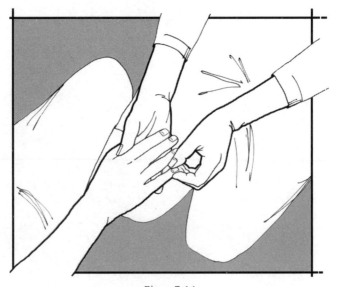

*Figure 7.14*

Any and all of the points on the fingertips are very sensitive. To connect at these points, just hold them gently one at a time. Stay with a point for one to three minutes; you may or may not be able to do all five fingertips, depending on time and circumstance. Watch the receiver's face or breathing; maintain eye contact if you can. Have no expectation, but be open to what the energy may bring. Sometimes the wordless exchange may feel like a dream, and begin with an image.

**9. Finish the arm and hand by repeating the light, feathery strokes from the shoulder down to the fingertips**

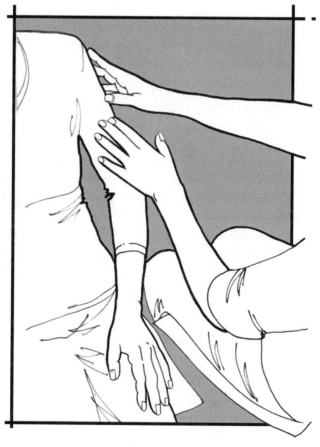

*Figure 7.15*

**10. Go to the receiver's other side**
Repeat steps 1–9 on the second hand, if possible.

**11. Finish**
When you are done, pause for a moment, and then consciously break contact with the receiver. Breathe out and relax. Observe the receiver. Notice any changes that may have occurred. Observe yourself, how do you feel? The final step is washing your hands again.

## WHEN SHARING TOUCH: WASH YOUR HANDS FIRST

Hand washing, necessary before you begin, can be a way to take a few moments to gather your thoughts. You can use it as a reminder to slow down, be present in your body, and be ready to connect through the senses. Perhaps when you stop at the sink you can let the sound of the running water remind you of a connection to nature. Healthcare practitioners often sing short songs to ensure they spend adequate time when washing their hands.

The following guidelines from the Center for Disease Control and Prevention (2010) and the World Health Organization (2009a, b), when done mindfully, can bring outer and inner practices together.

### Hand washing guidelines

1. Wet hands with water.

2. Apply enough soap to cover all hand surfaces.

3. Rub hands palm to palm in a circular manner.

4. Place the right palm over the back of the left hand and interlace the fingers and rub forward and backward.

5. Place the left palm over the back of the right hand and interlace the fingers and rub forward and backward.

6. Place the palms together with fingers interlaced and rub back and forward.

7. Place the backs of the fingers in the palms of the opposite hand, interlock the fingers and rub the fingertips back and forward.

8. Clasp the left thumb in the right palm and rotate.

9. Clasp the right thumb in the left palm and rotate.

10. Rub the tips of the right fingers on the palm of the left hand.

11. Rub the tips of the left fingers on the palm of the right hand.

12. Rinse the hands with water.

13. Dry the hands thoroughly with a paper towel.

14. Turn off the faucet with the used paper towel.

15. Your hands are now clean!

A hand sanitizer may be used only when the hands are not visibly soiled. The giver should bear in mind that hand sanitizers may cause dermatitis and dryness on the hands and may affect the quality of the massage. After applying the hand sanitizer, follow steps 3 to 11 of the hand washing instructions and allow your hands to air dry completely.

## The inner practice: Both
### Movement and stillness have value

When you are at a meridian point you may wonder what you will do in such a limited space. In France, acupressure is called 'micro-massage', which indicates that the approach to a meridian point is small, usually involving the fingertips. With the fingertip stationary, the practitioner can make a rotating motion, use intermittent pressure, or just hold a point. It depends on the location of the point and what is appropriate for the receiver. For those receiving comforting touch, just holding the point in a way that feels connected will suffice to provide benefits.

When you chose to hold a point it does a number of things. It creates some stillness in the sequence. While movement during a massage supports the more active, conscious functions of the body, stillness supports the receptive, sub-conscious activity. Both are important. For the giver, holding a meridian point is an opportunity to breathe out, drop your shoulders, and soften your arms and upper body. Remember, touch carries information as well as sensation, so your relaxation will be communicated to the receiver.

Attempt to be at a point for at least one minute, or up to three minutes. Your guiding principle is to be receiver-centered, so whatever the receiver can tolerate is a key factor. If you do not have enough time to work with all of the points, it is better to make a selection. Let your centered awareness guide you to what feels 'best' at the moment. Perhaps the receiver has symptoms that may be addressed with the meridian points that you select.

If your mind is too active, and you need another way to focus, you can add imagination (part of your spirit) to the process. As you hold a point, imagine that your fingertip emits a beam of light. Shine this beam of light into the point. *Reminder:* This is not a lengthy process, just a few seconds. When you stop, see and feel what happens. Observe the receiver's breathing, their face, and any changes in the muscles.

Observe yourself. This is one of the ways that sharing touch can benefit the giver. Bringing together the physical (through touch) and the awareness (through observing) will also engage the energetic, revealing the wholistic nature of your being.

Chapter 9

# At a Glance

## The Sequence and Reminders

After you have practiced the gentle hand massage detailed in Chapter 8, you can use this reference as a guide when you are providing it for someone. Remember the preliminary steps described in Chapters 6 and 7: consider the receiver's current condition, be aware of cautions or contraindications, consult with the health professional in charge of the care plan, and gather any needed supplies.

Spend at least three to five minutes on a hand; up to about 15 minutes; the total sequence should take no more than 20–30 minutes. Vary the protocol as needed to accommodate the receiver, yourself and the environment.

**Preparation**

1.  *Wash your hands* thoroughly with soap and water.

2.  Approach the receiver with respect.

3.  Breathe out slowly three times to bring your awareness and body together.

4.  If necessary, warm your hands by rubbing them briskly together.

5.  Tell the receiver what you are going to do and ask for permission to proceed. Make the receiver comfortable and then make yourself comfortable in either a seated or standing position.

**First contact says hello**

6.  Look at the receiver's hands to *evaluate* his or her individual needs. Avoid areas as necessary as described in Chapter 6 'Before You Begin'.

7.  Use both hands to make *feathery strokes* down the arm, from shoulder to fingertips. Repeat a few times.

**Bring warmth to the connection**

8.  Provide a sense of support by resting one of your hands on the receiver's arm. With your other hand make gentle, *warming circles* around the shoulder joint.

9.  Use one hand to make warming circles around the elbow.

10. Place the receiver's wrist between your palms, one on top, and one underneath. Gently make warming circles across the top of the wrist.

11. Support the receiver's hand with palm down. Use your top hand to make gentle circles over the knuckles.

**Stroke the hand to generate flow**

12. With the receiver's palm down, *stroke the top of the hand* with your thumbs, as if smoothing open the pages of a book, from the center out to the sides. Stroke at the top, center and bottom of the hand a few times in each area. This area is not well padded, and should be stroked lightly.

13. If possible, turn the receiver's hand over with their palm facing up. Use gentle *gliding strokes across the palm* in the same sequence from top to bottom described in step 12.

14. With the palm either up or down, *stroke the fingers* from knuckle to fingertip. Use any one or combination of the following: small circles, 'walking', gliding. Do not squeeze the fingers. Become aware of the temperature of the fingers as you stroke them.

15. Check in with the receiver, by asking or observing, to make sure the strokes and the pressure are comfortable for them.

**Maintain the connection**

16. Hold, gently press or massage any or all of the following points:

    ◦ LI 4 between the thumb and index finger (*Note*: Do not use in pregnancy.)

    ◦ PC 6 on the inner arm near the wrist.

    ◦ PC 8 on the palm.

    ◦ SI 3 behind the knuckle of the pinky finger, at the border of the light and dark skin.

    ◦ TW 4 on the back of hand at the wrist crease.

    ◦ Points at fingertips at the base of the nails. Hold each finger in turn, if time allows, otherwise chose to focus on one or more fingers.

**Complete one hand**

17. Finish one hand by using the same *light, feathery stroke* that you started with, going from the shoulder down to the fingertips, repeating it a few times.

18. Go to the *other hand*, and follow steps 6 through 17.

**Finishing**

19. When you feel you are done, *thank the receiver*.

20. You might *sit quietly* for a few moments to observe how your shared experience has affected both of you.

21. *Wash your hands* thoroughly when finished.

## THE INNER PRACTICE: INCORPORATE IT INTO YOUR DAY

Once you are aware of touch as a means of communication, you can use it as an activity to share, but you can also bring bits of it into daily life. For instance, when tasks have to get done, and a caregiver feels pressed for time, it can be easy to become frustrated when someone resists. Parts of the touch sequence have come in handy at times like that.

The light, feathery stroking of the arm can help orient someone in space, for instance, which can be calming. A caregiver found this technique to be useful with a woman with dementia who awoke with agitation and was too upset to cooperate with getting dressed. When words couldn't coax her to calmness, the caregiver found that using several soothing strokes down the arm helped the woman regain her composure. It was also used with a man with dementia when he resisted being shaved. The caregiver did not get into a struggle with him, but instead used soothing strokes as a way to smooth the transition and allow her to perform the task.

In the midst of routine care, a hand placed on the shoulder, accompanied perhaps by an encouraging exhalation, can be a meaningful experience. JD Elder, coordinator of the Massage Therapy Program at Mount Sinai Medical Center in New York, says the hospital will be opening a new palliative care unit that will provide services for patients, caregivers and staff. 'We plan to have workshops for nurses and patient care associates to be sure they are exposed to our perspective,' he explained. 'Though they may not be offering a hand massage, when they provide other types of physical care, like taking blood pressure, they can approach those tasks with the same kind of consideration and presence. We try to teach them that in the process of taking the blood pressure they can rest their hand mindfully on someone's shoulder for a moment. That will give a small dose of reassurance, as opposed to just throwing on the cuff, taking the reading and walking away.

'The speed of what one does sets the tone for the message we convey. As professionals, that is where our level of awareness and self-control is important,' he added. 'It is our ability to interact mindfully, slowly and quietly, putting aside for a moment the million things we may have to do, in order to be more present for the time that we share with our patients.'

Some caregivers have found the meridian points useful for self-care. They have, for instance, found the Large Intestine 4 point to be helpful with headaches. When using a single point for something like that, touch can be applied to it frequently throughout the day.

# *Part 3*

# The Reality of Practicing

Chapter 10

# Ten Challenges to Sharing Touch

At times in life we have to embark on a journey we might not otherwise want to take—whether it's an illness, accident or frailness as we age. We are meant to undertake this journey, but it is only natural that there may be some resistance. Even someone who wants only to provide comforting touch may find they need courage, camaraderie and a little nudge to take the first step. Though you may have the best of intentions, sharing touch, even with those you love, may not always be easy. What are some of the challenges?

## 1. Slowing down

When do you think this passage was written?

> In the past, people practiced...the principle of balance. They ate a balanced diet at regular times, arose and retired at regular hours, avoided overstressing their bodies and minds, and refrained from overindulgence of all kinds...These days, people have changed their way of life. They drink wine as though it were water, indulge excessively in destructive activities...They do not know the secret of conserving their energy and vitality. Seeking emotional excitement and momentary pleasures, people disregard the natural rhythm and order of the universe. They fail to regulate their lifestyle and diet, and sleep improperly. (Ni 1995, p.1)

This complaint comes from *The Yellow Emperor's Classic*, a basic text of Chinese medicine that appeared around 2000 years ago. Apparently, stress is not new, and every generation has its challenges to tranquility and carefree living.

Slowing down was never easy for average human beings who are busy with learning, working, and raising a family. Even back in the day, meditation was compared to the effort of sitting in the middle of a rushing stream. Today, accelerated transportation, high-speed communication and crowded living all contribute to our sense of an increased pace. Slowing down in the midst of it all may be a difficult, almost unnatural gesture. It is a challenge you will most likely face, one that may take repeated attempts to overcome. Like meditation, switching gears to a slower inner pace takes *practice*.

Do not equate slowness or stillness with doing nothing. Slowing down is not a matter of doing less, but of feeling more. 'A body at peace is not still; rather its flow of excitation is like that of a big river—deep and full' (Lowen 1990, p.168). This provides the giver as well as the receiver with the opportunity for greater sharing.

## 2. It is hard to be soft

We are often so busy that we do not realize how tense our muscles have become, and consequently how much sensitivity we sacrifice. Sharing touch invites you to pause, to allow you to use your fingers to 'listen', picking up sensations that can become guidance. You touch and let yourself be touched in return.

As your senses come alive, you begin to remember, 'I am a body. My body is soft, everything is flowing, and my breath brings in life.' This is pleasure, yes, but also the basis of morality. It is from awareness of our own humanness that we can respect and love others.

Let your touch be easy, soft. Let it be a reprieve from all that is harsh and fast. Soften for the times when you need to be soft, so you will remember how to love. When you don't know what to say, or perhaps someone doesn't want to listen, or words just aren't enough, you can let your love flow, more strongly than you know, through your hands.

## 3. There could be resistance

Some people have an aversion to touch, for any number of possible reasons. The meaning of touch for a receiver derives from earlier encounters, the goals for the touch experience, cultural factors and family history. The elderly or ill may also experience changes in body image, making them more or less accepting of touch (Hollinger and Buschmann 1993). If they have a great need for privacy or are very territorial, they may not be receptive to being touched in a sustained way.

For those challenged by dementia, their perception of touch may amount to a confused misunderstanding of what you are sharing. In these circumstances you will see in their eyes and their facial expression that they are misinterpreting the touch you are offering. Moving cautiously, gently and with reassurance will help to alleviate the distress that they are feeling; however, you may not be able to impact their level of understanding and consequently, may not be able to share touch while they are in this state of mind. A good diversion or mood changer is to tell stories, reminisce or sing songs, which can be a helpful preface to touch and helps to create a positive state of mind.

If the receiver declines touch—either through a verbal statement or a non-verbal gesture—their desire should be honored, as it is more important than your intention. If you find yourself with a recipient who is not interested in receiving therapeutic touch, or for whom touch is not practical, there are some suggestions for alternative paths you might consider pursuing in Chapter 6 'Before You Begin'.

Sometimes, however, the giver will resist. You will say, 'I don't have time.' However, it may be that you're tired or upset, or you do not feel well yourself. Acknowledge your own feelings and needs as an important part of learning to trust yourself. Don't resist resistance, whether it comes from the receiver, or from within you.

## 4. Dealing with fear

Having awareness of fears and facing them is important to caregivers. Fear and denial of the distress related to caregiving can prevent us from being gentle and from providing appropriate help. Caregivers sometimes inadvertently fail to provide the best care due to these unchallenged fears. Examples of this might include encouraging continuation with a medical treatment despite knowing that it offers no benefit, or failing to provide treatment for pain and symptoms because of fear or a negative belief about the treatment, its meaning or effect.

In his book *Smile at Fear*, meditation teacher Chogyan Trungpa describes a peaceful way to embrace this basic emotion. The first step is simply to admit it when we feel fearful. This admission, he says, is accompanied by a feeling of tenderness and sadness, along with self-acceptance. 'When that kind of friendliness to oneself occurs, then one also develops friendliness toward the rest of the world,' he writes (Trungpa 2009, p.36).

Because using touch mindfully brings body and mind together, it can be a kind of meditation in action. Through a mindful practice, challenges in life become opportunities to put our intentions to be loving into action. Our genuine attempts, whether fully achieved or not, help remind us of our own goodness and the goodness in all life. Basic goodness is something we all experience, but may not take the time to savor. 'Whenever you see a bright and beautiful color, you are witnessing your own inherent goodness,' Mr. Trungpa continues:

> whenever you taste something sweet or sour, you are experiencing your own basic goodness. If you are in a room and you open the door and walk outside, there is a sudden breeze of fresh air. Such an experience may last only a second, but that whiff of fresh air is the smell of basic goodness. (Trungpa 2009, p.9)

This sense of connection is not an abstract idea, but a felt experience. It includes a feeling of being in sync with one's self and with others, and a sense that everything is proceeding as it should. You accept the risks and responsibilities of your actions; you are ready to defend your stance. With a body–mind response to challenges you may feel less alone and more connected to each other and to deeper sources of life.

## 5. 'Nothing' seems to be happening

It's common to have questions about the effects of your touch. We often look for clues and reassurance from external sources. Such behaviors include asking for feedback about the effects of our touch, asking for the receiver's opinion about it, trying to read the receiver's facial expression or behavior. Signs of comfort and relaxation, statements affirming positive effects and behaviors that indicate effect can be validations that something is happening through the massage.

However, if no feedback is forthcoming, either positive or negative, we tend to think 'nothing' happened, nothing worked, or the massage was not effective. When the receiver has communication barriers, this is especially difficult because we are compelled to read other signs and behaviors rather than verbal communication that is reliable or has meaning.

One of the hardest things to learn is to attach value and, as a result, feel comfortable with our own inner thoughts and perceptions about the work that we are doing. Feeling confident about the massage and how we share massage is an important aspect of comfort for the caregiver. The caregiver should do the hand massage to the best of their ability and within the limits of what the receiver can accept. The caregiver can assume that their effort was beneficial if it met the needs of the receiver and achieved the goals of care. This feeling of confidence comes with practice and experience, knowledge of the benefits and effects, and of how to modify massage to best suit the receiver. Working with a mentor or peers can also provide the feedback that helps to validate good practice. However, confidence and comfort in good practice comes from within and can be supported through self-awareness, preparation and inner practices that are discussed throughout this book.

## 6. Sharing touch can feel awkward at first

Although touch is a natural instinct, using it in a deliberate way doesn't always come automatically. In fact, we often feel awkward and inexperienced when we first start to use touch with a new awareness. Having a teacher on site is a wonderful way to overcome any initial hesitation. Many facilities have integrative medicine services, so a massage therapist may be available. Nurses and nursing assistants also often have training in massage, therapeutic touch or energetic practices like Reiki. See if you can find someone to demonstrate and support you.

Try not to take yourself too seriously as you learn. We all remember fondly the awkward moments, conversations and actions in the past, and while we would like to change some of those moments, they helped to create the wise and knowing practice that is now part of our essence.

JD Elder, the massage therapy coordinator at Mount Sinai Medical Center's Hertzberg Palliative Care Institute, tells caregivers, 'We are all "beginners at the beginning" and this awareness helps us to remain alert to the potential novelty or newness in every massage encounter.' If caregivers take an interest in what he's doing, he teaches them basic foot massage and hand massage. 'I try to show them how to gently use their hands, to apply light massage pressure and that even if it seems like they're doing "nothing" it can be helpful. Touching someone with the intent to comfort, as well as to connect with empathy and compassion, makes a great deal of difference to the perceived quality of the experience,' he says. The integrative team at Mt. Sinai offers massage therapy free of charge, for both the patient and the family.

## 7. The receiver may become emotional

One of the greatest benefits of a focused, gentle use of touch is that it evokes a relaxation response. As the body and mind relax, the muscles will release, and as a result a person might let go of some pent-up emotions. In a massage therapy relationship, there is often a strong bond between the giver and receiver that transcends usual acquaintances, friendships and relationships. The effects of massage often become a highlight of the receiver's life with which no other relationship can compare. With massage, a powerful hormone called oxytocin is also released. This hormone is responsible for increasing relaxation, reducing blood pressure and alleviating anxiety (Uvnäs-Moberg 2003). Positive interactions created during a touch experience, plus the release of oxytocin and resulting positive physiological effects help to prime the receiver for an emotional release. The giver's awareness of this further enhances the bond with the receiver, and creates added meaning.

Emotional releases often take the form of tears. The giver may experience distress or discomfort when there is an emotional release and may often become emotional themselves. How comfortable are you when people cry or tell you that they are upset? Are you able to identify and offer support, or do you feel awkward and unable to react in a comforting way? Making sure that the receiver knows that they are in a safe, supportive environment is very important. With people who are ill or approaching the end of their life, emotional releases are very common and are usually about loss, love and emotional pain or suffering. During some studies, recipients sometimes released feelings of anger or frustration about their situation.

Should a receiver become emotional, you can pause in what you are doing and show that you are aware that they are upset and that you are concerned. You can ask the receiver if they would like you to resume your massage or if they would prefer that you stop for a while, giving them a chance to process their feelings. If strong emotions come up and the receiver might benefit from counseling or pastoral care, you can let the person in charge of the healthcare plan know.

## 8. Changes in the environment

Practitioners note that the time of day, as well as the time of year, can affect their work. Towards the end of winter, participants learning the hand massage, as well as the therapists supervising them, all had a difficult time: people seemed tired, making appointments for supervision was difficult, and no one seemed to be getting good results. The energy of winter, or lack of it, affected everyone. Knowing that the life force is constantly moving, the group held on together for a couple of weeks until the mood shifted and a better energy flow returned as spring began.

Whether you are a morning person or a night person may also affect you. The time, season and surroundings all contribute to your physical, energetic and mental state, so don't expect to feel the same every time you attempt to share comforting touch. Having said that, if there are particular self-care activities that help to improve your disposition at times when you are not feeling your best, give them a try.

## 9. You are tired

It is common to tire more easily during the winter, especially at the end of the winter, when we have been using energy reserves to stay warm and muscles may be tight from bracing against the cold. Overwork, worry and age will also affect our reserves of energy. The philosopher-physicians of Chinese medicine consider personal energy, or *Qi*, one of the three treasures of life, along with mind/spirit (*Shen*) and essence (*Jing*). As valuable resources, these three elements are to be used conservatively, as their interaction is what constitutes health, happiness, stability and mental clarity.

So when you feel tired, do not overextend yourself and feel you have to 'perform' a massage. Accept how you feel. Find a way to restore yourself first, whether it is through a nap, an inner practice, or using some of the meridian points for fatigue on yourself. Maybe you can get together with a friend or family member to practice the hand massage on each other, as a way to both learn and feel cared for.

## 10. You need to create a team

All of the experiences described in this book were the result of a team approach to care. Find support from local practitioners— whether the physician, nursing staff, social worker, psychologist, physical therapist, massage therapist or acupuncturist—before undertaking the use of a hand massage. You may not be aware of contraindications or cautions that need to be taken, but they will be. Everyone's situation is different and guidelines may change; they will be able to answer questions that may come up.

Professionals rely on team members too. JD Elder is very grateful for input from other practitioners:

> When working with someone who is seriously ill, being sick is only one aspect of the problem. There may be many other factors contributing to a patient's discomfort. For example, a bed may be uncomfortable, or the patient's skin may be itchy. Perhaps the noise or the lighting in the environment might be bothering them. There is also the emotional distress of a patient and their loved ones. Patients are often worried about their own well-being as well as whether their family is alright.
>
> How one offers a massage can help to peel away at least *some* of these variables. We can adjust and monitor the environment prior to the session (e.g. dim the lights, put on music and use prescribed lotions to soothe dry, irritated skin). We can also importantly provide a soothing massage and thereby help to reduce stress and distressing symptoms, thoughts and emotions. However, to fully expand our ability to help our patients, we must acknowledge that we cannot do it all and we need to refer to other team members or clinicians when necessary—for example, a chaplain, psychologist or social worker who can provide much needed additional support. That is the benefit of an integrative approach to patient care—we rely on each other's expertise, and our collaboration is in the best interest of the patient.

When you meet a challenge, don't think of it as a problem; see it as what is true in the moment. Every time you share your touch it will be different. Experiences will change according to the seasons of the day, as well as the year. Your own strength and courage will vary. The receiver's interest may be evident or not. Nothing stays the same. What is important is following the flow, allowing enough freedom in the session for something unique to happen, something genuine, between you and the receiver.

# When sharing touch:
# Don't resist resistance

John was a devoted husband. His love for his wife, Christine, was palpable and profound. Sadly, she was in the end stages of cancer and had trouble with fatigue, pain and anxiety. John was very vigilant and managed all her care, including the people who provided homecare services to his wife. His training in the military gave him a very structured way to handle all the daily arrangements. John had no other outlet to share the anxiety that he felt, so he poured his distress into vigilantly managing Christine's schedule: mealtimes, medication times, exercises, home health aide visits, daily washing, social worker and nurse visits. He felt he had control over the situation when he did this; however, the people who were caring for Christine at times experienced a regimented and inflexible man.

Managing Christine's schedule gave John a sense of control even though her health was out of control. It alleviated some of the anxiety that he felt since he was not the type of man to talk freely about the pain he felt and the possibility of losing the love of his life. His philosophy was that he needed to stay strong and take control of everything that would relieve Christine of any burden.

One day the nurse called to schedule Christine's weekly visit. John told the nurse 'Come at 2.30! That way, Christine will have finished her lunch and had a chance to rest.' The nurse arrived at 2.45. John was in another room when the home health aide let the nurse in to see Christine. Upon seeing the nurse tending to Christine, John stood in the doorway and flew into a rage, shouting at the nurse 'You're late! What time do you think this is to arrive to take care of my wife? I told you to come at 2.30.'

The nurse immediately became fearful since John's anger was intense. She immediately thought: He's blocking the doorway and I'm trapped in this room if he continues to be this angry. She also thought and felt: He must be really stressed out taking care of his wife. She felt concern and compassion for the pain he must be feeling.

She took a deep breath and said, 'I don't know if you realize it, but you are shouting at me and blocking the doorway, which is making me a little scared. I might need to leave and come back later when you are not so upset.' The nurse could see that John's anger was lessening as he realized how his anger was affecting her. She continued. 'You are doing a great job managing everything for your wife. I'm so amazed at how well you take care of her. It must be very hard for you when things don't always go the way you want them to. I'm here to help you and only want the best for you and Christine. I'm sorry if I did not get here at the time you needed me to. There are many things that hold us up out there.'

Upon hearing this, John offered his apologies and told the nurse that he didn't realize that he was so angry that he scared her. He loved every nurse that ever took care of his wife and would never want to hurt them. The nurse could see that he was overwhelmed with emotion and reached out to hold his hand and offer her support and compassion through touch. This was a very meaningful moment between them and thereafter they were the best of friends.

## THE INNER PRACTICE:
## RETURNING TO THE CENTER

Life's rhythms include periods of activity and rest, light and dark, waxing and waning. The same principle of constant change will apply to the practice that involves 'centering' or calming your mind when you want to share touch with someone. Feeling centered is not a constant state, and returning to it is as much a part of the practice as attempting to create it.

As you center yourself before you begin a massage, you take a moment to assess your own inner environment and bring your thoughts and feelings to a place where you can focus on the receiver, so the touch will be 'receiver centered'. You may apply the inner practices—such as breathing, meditation or visualizations—to help bring about a sense of calm. Yet there are many times when this may feel particularly difficult due either to your own feelings or to the behavior of the receiver.

Many times people who have chronic illness or dementia, or are at the end stages of a disease process, are not happy; sometimes they will lash out at you. As a result, you may become angry or upset and not feel like reaching out to touch that person. Using tools that you find helpful to manage your mood is recommended at these times, whether it is one of the suggested inner practices or taking a break to do something you enjoy, such as going for a walk, listening to music, or doing a craft. Sometimes sitting with the negative thoughts and feelings and waiting for them to go away is also helpful.

Bringing your awareness to your mood and the quality of the thoughts that you are having before you touch is an important preparation exercise that is an essential part of the massage. When you are nervous, your hands may shake, you may stutter, or you may feel and act awkwardly. When you are angry, your touch may be short and abrupt. When you are happy, your touch may be energetic and light. When you share a hand massage with someone, your thoughts will be communicated by the way you move: your speed, pressure, sensitivity and the length of time you give it.

If you cannot be neutral in your approach, or don't feel particularly calm, you might try the use of a technique called 'unconditional positive regard'. Unconditional positive regard is a term coined by Carl Rogers, an influential psychologist and founder of the humanist approach to psychology. It is a way of showing acceptance and support for a person despite what may be their negative behaviors.

This would involve focusing your thoughts on a declaration such as, 'I want the best for _____[the name of the person]'. Then integrate the meaning of the sentence so that you have an emotional connection to the statement and as a result to the person. You have successfully integrated the meaning into your practice when you understand what the person's needs are that are causing them to act in a negative way and can feel compassion for them. Once you have this awareness, you can then tailor your approach to meeting their needs as best you can. Wait until you feel the positive emotion towards the person before sharing touch.

In sharing a hand massage with someone, you don't want to create negative feelings in the course of the experience. By showing unconditional positive regard you focus on cultivating an inner state that helps to ensure that you and the receiver share a good experience. This is an important way of thinking, since we all, at some point, have negative thoughts about ourselves and others. Negativity leads to judgments that often change the way we interact with people and interfere with our ability to connect.

You may not always be successful in thinking positive thoughts about the person, however, and in those moments sharing a hand massage may not be the best option. On the other hand, sometimes the act of providing the massage and the positive feelings that it can bring will create the beneficial changes you need. Returning to your center means actively managing your thoughts and emotions—in whatever way you choose to do it—so that when you reach out you will extend your inner beauty through your hands.

Chapter 11

# Adapting for Different Needs

The hands are the easiest, safest and most natural places to share touch, however, using massage with someone who is elderly or ill may require some modifications. There are occasions when sharing a hand massage should be avoided or when the giver should exercise caution. Cautions and contraindications are addressed in Chapter 6 'Before You Begin', along with alternative therapies that might be used in place of massage therapy.

## Common illnesses in the elderly

When illnesses have progressed to later stages, the symptoms of disease may impact all activities of daily living. At any time when the person receiving massage reports discomfort, or is bothered by symptoms of their illness, massage is no longer appropriate and treating the symptoms becomes a priority. Listed below are the most common illnesses that affect the elderly and some guidelines on your massage practice. Bear in mind that touch is almost always possible in some form or other.

### Dementia

Dementia is an irreversible debilitating disease that results from loss of brain function over time. People with dementia gradually experience loss of memory, language, personality, perceptive and cognitive skills. They can no longer perform the usual tasks on a daily basis that we all take for granted. In the advanced stage, because of their immobility, they may lose muscle function, with their arms and legs becoming hypertonic with deformities referred to as contractures. People with dementia often reside in nursing homes as a result of the intensity of caregiving that is required.

As these people lose their ability to speak and connect verbally, touch becomes a significant way to communicate with them. Many studies have been conducted using various forms of touch that support its usefulness in addressing the unique concerns of people with dementia. Studies and experience show that massage is accepted quite readily by this population (Malaquin-Pavan 1997; Trombley 2003). Tender touch used in a one-year demonstration project found it could alleviate anxiety and decrease pain (Sansone and Schmitt 2000). Hand massage has been shown to decrease agitated behavior (Hicks-Moore and Robinson 2008; Kramer and Smith 1999; Remington 2002) in people with dementia. Following a hand massage, caregivers have found that recipients improved in functional abilities and they were more alert (Kilstoff and Chenoweth 1998).

Suggestions and stories about adapting a hand massage for someone with dementia are provided throughout this book. People with dementia usually welcome touch when approached slowly and with genuine concern. Challenges occur when they are wandering or engaging in agitated activities. They may shout, cry or pull away, looking at you through confused eyes. Verbal instructions may not be of value at times like that, but you can try using touch to communicate. A mindful gesture on the shoulder or arm may help. Bear in mind that repetitive movements are often comforting and predictable and offer the most soothing touch experience for people with dementia. Use a little bit at a time to start, if necessary, and gradually build on what you can do.

If you do use words to try to placate them, imagine your voice is a soothing hand. If they ask questions repeatedly, guide their attention to what you are doing; ask them how the touch feels, name the fingers as you touch them, or count the fingers. If they pull away and seem uncooperative, stop the massage and offer reassurance. Try another approach or come back another time. Most of all, be patient. Of all the people with whom you can share massage, those with dementia can reap great benefits from its non-verbal, yet deeply personal exchange, one that can sometimes allow the caregiver a glimpse of the person they once were.

## Cancer

While a gentle hand massage is a safe type of massage therapy to offer people with cancer, you may still need to make adjustments in what you do and how long you do it, based on how the person is feeling, the symptoms affecting them and the treatment that they are receiving for the cancer. The physician and healthcare team will determine whether massage is appropriate and they must always be consulted prior to using massage.

Cancer affects people differently depending on the type of cancer, the extent of the disease and the organs and systems that are affected. In general, most types of cancer cause weakness, fatigue, malaise and weight loss. Cancer affecting the lungs will cause shortness of breath and a cough. Cancers of the blood, such as leukemia, will affect blood counts and cause susceptibility to bleeding, anemia and infections. Cancer in the abdomen, such as colon cancer or pancreatic cancer, may cause pain, cramps, diarrhea or constipation. Bone cancer causes bone pain, a dull insidious constant ache. Liver cancer will cause pain and swelling in the abdomen and when blocking the bile duct, will cause jaundice. Brain cancer may cause mental status changes, seizures and other neurological problems depending on where the brain tumors are located.

You may notice 'cachexia', the wasting of tissue and muscles, which is described in the 'Cautions and contraindications' section of Chapter 6. A lack of connective or fatty tissue supporting the muscles and bones in the hands and arms will affect how you do the massage, emphasizing a need for very light, gentle strokes.

When cancer is at the end stage and has spread to other organs and tissues (metastases) and the person affected is approaching the end of life, massage to the hands is very comforting and a wonderful protocol for caregivers to use. Use light touch and soft, slow massage therapy strokes. Lotions and creams will be helpful to the skin that is often dry and papery; use whatever is approved by the facility if the receiver is institutionalized. Check with the receiver often to make sure they are positioned comfortably and the strokes are not too deep or causing pain.

Massage for people with cancer is used and taught in leading healthcare facilities in New York City. Wendy Miner has been program coordinator at the Integrative Medicine Service (IMS) at Memorial Sloan-Kettering Cancer Center where massage therapy and practice protocols are developed to meet the needs of acutely ill cancer patients undergoing treatment. (See the 'When sharing touch' box at the end of this chapter.) At Mount Sinai Medical Center, JD Elder coordinates the massage therapy program that offers comforting massage to cancer patients and others as part of the hospital's Hertzberg Palliative Care Institute. At Beth Israel Medical Center, the inpatient MJHS Hospice and Palliative Care unit, under the guidance of chief medical officer Russell Portenoy, integrates standard pain management protocols that are further supported by massage therapy, offered by both licensed massage therapists and supervised massage therapy students.

## Stroke

A stroke is caused when arteries supplying blood to the brain become blocked, causing an ischemic stroke, or rupture, causing a hemorrhagic stroke. Areas of the brain are deprived of oxygenated blood as a result of interruption to the blood flow or bleeding into the tissues. The tissues affected start to die and, in turn, affect the body functions governed by that area of the brain. Depending on the area affected, the person may no longer be able to move the muscles on one side of their body, or walk, talk, see or feel things in a normal way.

Strokes affecting the right side of the brain will cause left side paralysis, vision problems, agitation and memory loss. Strokes affecting the left side of the brain will cause right side paralysis, speech and language problems, slow behavior and memory loss.

Spastic or flaccid paralysis will be the result, depending on the motor neurons affected. The arm and hand on the unaffected side will look and feel completely different compared to the affected side.

When sharing massage with someone who has flaccid paralysis on one side, be sure the hand, wrist and elbow are in a position of comfort. With spastic paralysis, you will find that movement is limited due to contractures and you will be performing massage in whatever position you find the arm. The person will not be able to move the affected arm or pull it away if the massage strokes are uncomfortable. As a result, the depth, strokes and pressure should be applied conservatively and you should ask the receiver for feedback as you work.

During the massage, you will need to support the arm consistently using pillows and bolsters. With spastic paralysis, if the hand is curled into a fist, the fingernails may break the skin on the palm of the hand. The primary caregiver will often place a rolled-up bandage, cotton ball or face towel in the hand to protect the palm from injury. As you work on the hand, do not try to force the fingers open, but work over the clenched hand. Over time, massage may help the muscles in the arm lengthen and increase movement.

## Heart disease

Heart disease affects a significant number of elderly people and may cause symptoms that will interfere with their comfort during massage. With advanced heart disease, the person may be short of breath at rest and require oxygen to assist their breathing. They may have a persistent cough and fluid on their lungs that causes congestion. Sometimes this congestion is audible when they breathe. When positioning a person with heart disease who is congested and short of breath, they must always be positioned with their chest elevated with a few pillows behind them. The oxygen should not be removed for massage. Some people with heart disease may have intermittent chest pain or palpitations. Chest pain is managed with the use of nitroglycerine, oxygen and rest. If chest pain occurs during the course of massage, you should stop and inform the facility staff or caregivers who will assist the person with taking medication and deciding on the next course of treatment. Massage may resume if the chest pain resolves and the receiver feels better.

People with heart disease may have swelling in their hands, feet and lower back. Because their heart is pumping inefficiently, fluid backs up into the lungs and the tissues. The easiest place for the fluid to settle is in the peripheries. If the person is bedbound, gravity sends the fluid to their hands and the base of their spine. If the person is ambulatory, you will see swelling in their feet, ankles and legs. Tissues that contain fluid may feel spongy to touch and look like an orange peel.

Swelling in the hands is easy to see. The hands and fingers look puffy and the shape of the hand is different. The swelling may result in rings and bracelets being too tight and the person may not be able to close their hand in a fist completely. Massage in this area must be very superficial if at all. You may, however, elevate the hand on a pillow so that gravity drains the fluid away from the hand. Consult with the healthcare practitioner before you proceed.

## Lung disease

Lung diseases include asthma, sarcoidosis, chronic obstructive airway disease or emphysema. Lung cancer may also cause symptoms that affect the ability to breathe. The area of lung tissue available to be used for breathing is minimal, so people with lung disease are short of breath even at rest and have a chronic cough that may produce phlegm. They will often be receiving oxygen: either by tubes under their nose or a mask covering their nose and mouth. Making people with breathing problems comfortable and positioning them in a way that their breathing is the best that it can be is important before starting massage. Any increased difficulty with breathing, coughing and wheezing will likely interrupt the massage.

Someone with lung disease should not be lying flat in bed, but should have their chest elevated on pillows. Prior to starting massage, a nebulizer treatment may be needed if the receiver is wheezing or there are high-pitched sounds when they breathe.

Wheezing is common with asthma and chronic airway obstruction. Nebulizer treatments open the airways and allow more air into the lungs. Certain nebulizers will cause tremors, so you should not be surprised if the receiver has a shake in their hand or has difficulty relaxing. Consult with the receiver, primary caregivers and facility staff where applicable regarding treatments needed if you are not involved with these decisions in general.

You may notice that the person's complexion is ashen, or that there is a blue or gray color to the skin. This is common in severe lung disease. Their nose may also be blue and the lips are sometimes blue or purple. While this color may be their baseline disposition, you should pay attention to whether the color changes during the course of the massage.

If the receiver becomes confused or agitated at any time, this may be a sign of poor oxygenation to the brain. You should discontinue the massage if this happens and inform the facility staff, caregivers or decision makers so they can decide on an appropriate treatment plan.

If the receiver has pneumonia or a chest infection, a common complication for people with lung disease, you will need to reschedule the massage as working on someone with an infection is contraindicated. You may also be at risk of exposure if the infection is spread through droplets in the air.

The skin on the hands and arms is often dry and discolored in someone with lung disease. You may notice blue nail beds or a gray or blue color to the fingertips caused by poor perfusion with oxygenated blood. People with lung disease are also cachectic, with limited connective tissue and fat stores under the skin. Areas with frail skin and no underlying fatty connective tissue should be massaged very lightly. When people with breathing problems relax, their breathing improves. You should not underestimate the value of hand massage in helping people with lung disease relax and feel better.

## Assessing symptoms

Whenever any symptom becomes bothersome to the receiver, the chance of achieving the desired effect of massage is reduced or lost. The receiver cannot relax if they are in pain. Similarly, they cannot concentrate on enjoying the massage if they are having difficulty breathing. They will not be able to tolerate massage when they are positioned in a way that is uncomfortable, and they will not benefit from the massage if the manner in which you are sharing massage causes pain or discomfort. Assessing the severity of symptoms is a helpful practice. It will guide you in deciding if you need to stop the massage, ask for assistance from other healthcare practitioners or whether a symptom may be helped through massage.

You may find it useful to use a scale to measure symptoms so you have an idea of how severe a receiver's symptoms are and whether these symptoms will interfere with massage or are helped by massage. A 0 to 10 pain scale is helpful to assess the severity of pain where the alert and oriented receiver can verbalize a number between 0 and 10 that correlates with the level of pain that they are experiencing, 0 correlating with no pain and 10 being the worst pain imaginable. A level of pain of 5 or above should cause you to enquire about pain management and collaborate with healthcare providers. The Wong-Baker FACES pain rating scale, which uses a picture of a face that corresponds with how they are feeling, can be useful for children and people who have communication or cognitive difficulties (Wong-Baker FACES Foundation 2011).

Similarly, there are assessment scales for anxiety, depression, shortness of breath, fatigue, nausea, insomnia and a host of other symptoms that may be valuable in quantifying the level at which the receiver is experiencing the symptoms. If you are working in a facility, the facility may have standardized scales that they use to assess the severity of symptoms.

Following massage, you may again assess the level of the symptoms experienced to evaluate if the receiver's experience has changed and whether the massage was helpful in reducing or alleviating the symptoms.

# Skin conditions

Rashes, redness, dry skin, cuts and bruises must be evaluated before massaging an area. You will need the physician's permission whenever there are skin problems.

Dry skin may be indicative of dehydration. If you pinch the skin lightly, pull up gently and then let go of the skin, you can see if skin tenting occurs. The elasticity and suppleness of the skin should bring the skin back to its normal position when you let go; however, if dehydrated, the skin will stay up in a tented position and return slowly to its normal position.

Dehydration occurs when the person is not able to stay adequately hydrated and may be accompanied by other symptoms, such as weakness, fatigue, cachexia, anorexia and weight loss. If the receiver has diarrhea, has not been eating or drinking enough or has been vomiting, they will most likely be dehydrated too. With dehydration, the receiver's blood pressure is expected to be low. Massage should be conservative using light, superficial strokes.

Bruises are painful to the touch and may be associated with swelling, heat and inflammation. If there are bruises on the hands and arms, these areas should be avoided during the hand protocol. You will need to adjust the pressure you apply if the person is prone to bruising too. The hand protocol may be shared if there are cuts on the hands and arms, but avoid massage directly over wounds, cuts and recent surgical sites.

Rashes that affect the entire area may prohibit the use of hand massage. There may be other areas in the body that are not affected by a rash where massage can be offered; however, massage in these areas are not addressed in this book. Depending on the type of rash and the treatment, the physician and healthcare team will be able to advise you about massage.

Rashes generally make the skin sensitive to touch and cause itchiness. The receiver should be encouraged not to scratch itchy skin as this causes injury and increases swelling and redness. It also makes the itchy area even itchier. Gentle tapping can offer relief in some cases, in addition to cold applications such as a cold, damp cloth.

# Hand disorders

When offering the hand massage protocol, in addition to the challenges of illness, there are unique situations affecting the arms and hands and impacting the massage that will also require adjustments to your approach.

Arthritis is the most common disorder affecting the hands. Rheumatoid arthritis causes inflammation, heat, redness and pain to the joints. In the acute phase of inflammation, the joints may be swollen and red, and massage cannot be done over the area. Movement of the fingers and joints may cause pain, and you may also see deformities in the joints. Your hand massage will need to be very light and superficial and guided by the receiver's reports of pain or discomfort. Make sure to support the hand and arm and minimize joint movement if it causes pain. It is best not to apply pressure on the bones and joints, which will also elicit pain if performed.

Contractures are another disorder that can affect the hands. A contracture is an abnormal shortening of muscles resulting in deformity in the area affected. Contractures most commonly affect the joints of the arms and legs and interfere with mobility. People who are bedbound or have brain and spinal cord problems frequently have contractures. It is often difficult to move and position the arms when they are affected by contractures. Do not attempt to pull the arm, wrist and hand straight or to force the arm into a position where it will not naturally stay. This may cause injury and pain.

With contractures, the hand massage protocol should be modified so you begin with the area that is easiest to access. This is most often the outer aspect of the arm, forearm, the back of the hand and thumb. Over the course of the massage, observe any small change that might occur. You should not expect the contracture to resolve completely over time since the causes are related to neurological damage in the brain, but you may find that with repeated gentle massage the muscles lengthen and release, with some movement in the area occurring more easily.

# Tubes and devices

When working in a healthcare setting, or working with someone who is ill and receiving medical treatment in their home, there are a number of medical devices that you may encounter. Many of these devices may not affect your ability to share a hand massage. You may, however, need to modify the positioning or your approach to massage based on the presence of medical devices. You should not be fearful about the presence of tubes and devices. If you are not sure about them, consult with the medical professionals before proceeding to find out how you may need to modify your massage.

## Intravenous lines

Intravenous catheters and lines are the most common medical equipment you will see on the hands and arms. They will have a dressing over the insertion site and be secured sometimes with sutures, and most often with a transparent dressing and tape. You must not massage over or close to an intravenous catheter. When working around intravenous lines, be mindful not to pull on or kink the tubing, disconnect the tubing or position pillows over the tubing. The receiver may be prescribed infusion therapies such as intravenous pain management, antibiotics, hydration, chemotherapy and nutritional supplements which they may be receiving continuously.

## AV graft

People with kidney disease who are receiving dialysis or who have received dialysis in the past may have an arterio-venous (AV) graft or fistula. This is a surgical procedure that connects arteries with veins in the arm to create a large vessel that can be accessed to filter the blood through a dialysis machine. If you touch the AV graft, you will be palpating large bulging vessels that buzz or vibrate under your fingers. This vibrating feeling represents the swirling or rushing of the arterial and venous blood together. Certain procedures are not permitted on the arm with an AV fistula such as blood specimen collection or taking blood pressure. You will need to contact the physician regarding permission to massage the hand and arm with an AV graft and you should not be surprised if you are not permitted to touch that arm.

## Urinary catheters and colostomy bags

Urinary catheters drain urine from the bladder. While you will not be working around catheters, the manner in which the receiver is positioned may impact the placement of catheter tubes and drainage bags. You should be aware of bags hanging from the side of the bed or chair making sure not to lean on or kink the tubing. Colostomy bags collect stool from a stoma in the abdomen, and are another area to be mindful to use caution around.

## Tracheostomy tubes

These are located in the throat and open the airway. When massaging the shoulder and arm, be careful not to pull on the tracheostomy ties that secure the tube in place. You will also need to be mindful about how the receiver is positioned so that their airway is open and they are breathing comfortably. On occasion, when people with tracheostomies cough, phlegm comes out of the tracheostomy tube. It may be necessary to stop the massage to allow them to remove the phlegm and clean up around the tube. If you routinely help with managing the tracheostomy, remember to wash your hands again before resuming the hand massage.

## Drainage tubes

Tubes of varying sizes are often used to reduce swelling, drain fluid from certain areas and collect the fluid in a drainage bag. Gravity removes the fluid from the area it is draining into a collection bag below the level of the affected area. You may see these devices in many areas of the body. If present, you should be mindful not to lean on or pull on these devices. Some drains operate using suction and so will not be affected by gravity. Pillows should not be placed where they will interfere with the drainage device.

Chest tubes will be located on the right or left side of the chest. These tubes cause a lot of pain and will interfere with the receiver's positioning for massage. The drainage device is often connected to a wall suction device which causes bubbling and a constant sound from the drainage device. You will need to pay particular attention to the receiver's breathing and their report of any pain during the massage. They should never be lying flat or on the chest tube. You will need to be mindful not to pull on or kink the tubing. Pillows can be used to support the arm over the chest tube but you should not apply pressure to or impede the drainage of fluid through the tube. People with chest tubes may also be receiving oxygen therapy.

## Monitoring devices

*Oxygen saturation monitors* are often attached to one of the fingers and monitor the oxygenation in the blood. The receiver will most likely be wearing an oxygen mask or tubing too. If the oxygen saturation reading is low, below 90 percent, the healthcare team may determine that a hand massage is not appropriate until the oxygen saturation level is higher.

*Blood pressure monitors* involve the application of a cuff to the arm that periodically takes the receiver's blood pressure. You may request one of the healthcare team members to remove the cuff from the arm so that you will be able to share a massage without interference from the blood pressure cuff. If this cannot be facilitated, periodic inflation of the blood pressure cuff will interrupt the massage. You should wait before continuing with the hand massage until the monitor has taken the blood pressure.

*Cardiac monitors* will have leads attached to the chest and in some instances, to the arms and legs. While sharing massage, make sure not to pull on or disconnect the leads. Lotion, if you use it, should also not be applied close to the leads, as it will interfere with the adherence of the pads. If the leads become detached, this will set off an alarm on the monitor and result in the facility staff needing to reattach or adjust the leads. You can work around the leads, being mindful not to interfere with their functioning. You may also see a screen that is recording the heart rhythm. It may be an interesting and useful activity to pay attention to the heart rate and rhythm at the start of the massage and to see if it changes throughout the massage. You most likely will see the heart rate slowing and the rhythm become more regular.

## Oxygen masks and tubes

These may be located over the nose and mouth. If you observe the receiver with an oxygen mask or nasal cannula, you should not remove it. The presence of oxygen therapy provides further information that the receiver has difficulty breathing and as a result, should not be positioned flat on the bed. Oxygen tubing should not interfere with the performance of hand massage but you will need to be mindful not to disconnect, pull on or kink the tubing. If you notice that the mask or tubing is not over the nose and/or mouth, ask the receiver if they need help to adjust it. If you are not routinely involved with adjusting the oxygen mask, ask the caregivers to help the receiver to position it correctly.

As with any new experience, there is a period of learning and adjustment. As you work around tubes and devices and learn about their functions, you will increase your level of comfort and proficiency at integrating them into a seamless massage practice.

## WHEN SHARING TOUCH: CONSIDER HELP FROM A CARING PROFESSIONAL

Touch Therapy for Caregivers is a class that has always been part of the Integrative Medicine Service (IMS) at Memorial Sloan-Kettering Cancer Center, one of the largest integrative medicine centers in the United States. Some 60 professionals at IMS work in research, education and treatment of symptoms associated with cancer and cancer treatment. Clinicians specializing in many disciplines—including massage therapy, music therapy, dance therapy, acupuncture, yoga, exercise, nutrition, and meditation—share their skills with thousands of people a year who are either outpatients or hospitalized. IMS aims to improve patient quality of life, manage symptoms, and provide education to healthcare professionals and the public, as well as conduct research in botanicals and clinical therapies that have potential benefits to cancer patients. As a service to patients, healthcare professionals and the general public, IMS has developed a website for people to learn more about their findings (Memorial Sloan-Kettering Cancer Center 2011).

Rocco Caputo, a licensed massage therapist and certified neuromuscular therapist, has been working for IMS for the past ten years. He has a lively, youthful demeanor and meets every visitor with a smile. In his massage therapy treatment room he balances the serious side of his work with a little playfulness.

Mr. Caputo teaches the class for caregivers once a month in the hospital's recreation room. The class is offered by IMS free of charge and is open to all who are interested in assisting loved ones going through cancer and cancer treatment. The 90-minute class usually begins with some attention to breathing.

'When someone is anxious they breathe in, but they often don't breathe out very well,' Mr. Caputo explained. 'I encourage the class participants to breathe in and then take a long, slow exhalation, attempting to empty the lungs completely, creating an empty void that should, upon the next inhale, allow fresh air to fill the void that had previously retained "old air".' He then provides instruction on how to use gentle touch, beginning with just placing one's hands on a receiver's shoulders, and then making soothing strokes over the upper back, arm or hand. Repetition and a light touch are a key.

'Gentle, caring, healing touch is an important thing to share. The studies show that simply holding hands can be valuable,' Mr. Caputo says, 'and we want people to receive the benefits that touch can provide.' Memorial Sloan-Kettering patients are referred to the IMS by medical staff for particular symptoms but are screened by the therapists before treatment begins to determine safety and appropriate ways to work.

The Integrative Medicine Service published a study in 2004 that looked at how massage, including light touch and foot massage, impacts symptoms associated with cancer and cancer treatment. Over a three-year period, 1290 patients took part, reporting symptom severity for pain, fatigue, stress/anxiety, nausea and depression. After receiving touch therapy, symptom scores were reduced by approximately 50 percent, with outpatients improving slightly more than inpatients (Cassileth and Vickers 2004).

Mr. Caputo knows that one of the initial problems he must address for caregivers is their fear. 'Far too many people stop touching their loved ones when treatment begins because they are afraid of all that's going on around them and fear doing the wrong thing,' he explained. 'The class teaches some of the technical aspects of touch, such as how to safely apply massage and to respect the equipment—the devices emerging from their loved ones—but not to be afraid of it.'

In his class, Mr. Caputo reviews contraindications and precautions used at Memorial Sloan-Kettering for cancer patients undergoing treatment: no massage over a recent incision site, radiation site or tumor. Steer clear of any tubes or devices. No massage below a lymph node dissection due to susceptibility for swelling (lymphedema) and no massage if there is a blood clot or platelet count below 50,000. (More on cautions and contraindications are included in Chapter 6 'Before You Begin'.)

'Taking the individual's situation into consideration, I will choose an area I can work on safely. Often it's just the hand due to plummeting platelet counts, a person's comfort, or many devices—tubes, stomach pegs, chest tubes, pumps, shunts—which may restrict work on other areas. But whatever area can be touched safely should be addressed.'

The professionals at Memorial Sloan-Kettering have found that when in an inpatient setting, 20 minutes is a good length of time for touch therapy. 'Our studies show that 20 minutes of inpatient massage has the same effect as a 60-minute massage as an outpatient or in a setting like a spa,' Mr. Caputo said. 'Twenty minutes turns out to be a long period of time in the hospital.' The best 'dosage' will be determined by the receiver's comfort, as well as the giver's ability. Two times a day for a few minutes may be better than one long massage weekly.

In addition to providing physical benefits, touch can provide a meaningful way for people to connect during a difficult time. 'It's a fact of life, though not a happy fact, that people's bodies break down,' Mr. Caputo reflected. 'You have the choice of how to be there for them. Lately, we're all on our communication devices—people text instead of touch—but touch is a wonderful way for people to make a real connection during such a time.'

Caregivers take on an overwhelming amount of varying tasks—paying bills, cleaning, cooking, running errands—much of which may go unsung. Lack of recognition sometimes makes the caregiver feel like they have to give more, eventually becoming exhausted. Mr. Caputo feels that providing a massage is a way to make your care tangible. 'If you spend a half hour providing a massage for your loved one, chances are it gets talked about,' he says, smiling and pretending to hold a phone to his ear. 'Your mother receives a call and she says, "Oh, my son just gave me a massage. I feel so much better!" It's something that stays with them, something you feel good about doing and is always appreciated. What's more, you can take some time afterward to reflect on what you felt during the experience. Maybe you can promise to take ten minutes for yourself afterwards, which could be a good self-care option.'

Though he would love to accompany caregivers back to the hospital room immediately following the class to give a private demonstration, there is almost never enough time after the class to provide one-on-one instruction. 'We have very full clinical schedules at the IMS, so it is rarely possible to go with a caregiver for an individual supervision,' he said. 'However, all the IMS massage therapists are willing to include caregiver instruction during an inpatient massage session; in the pediatric unit, parents are always encouraged to join in and receive a lesson in massage, unless they decline.'

His pediatric work focuses on relieving symptoms that are specific to pediatric cancers and its treatment, in addition to providing comfort care for end-stage children. All pediatric cancers are treated on the pediatric floor, and Mr. Caputo works most often with children affected by leukemias, neuroblastomas and osteosarcomas. 'Once a prognosis is made that the child has entered an actively dying stage, physical therapy and occupational therapy are discontinued,' he explained. 'Once that happens, they don't get much touch except for turning, procedural touch and parent interaction. In these cases I apply comfort care massage, to provide relaxation and comfort in the child's last days.

'Consent to provide touch therapy is received at the initial consultation with the parents. I explain exactly what I'm going to do, where and how massage will be applied,' Mr. Caputo said. 'Parents are given the option to watch, learn or participate. For very young children, I often massage the parent first. This lets the child see that everything is okay; the parent is happy and then the child feels it's safe to join in. I work with the parent, I work with the child, and the parent works with the child.'

Massage is becoming increasingly used for symptom relief for people with cancer, and many facilities now offer it as part of an integrative medicine service. If you are caring for someone with cancer, and want to explore the benefits of touch for alleviating symptoms, find out from your medical providers if their organization has integrative practitioners available or if they can help you find a qualified practitioner. The 'Resources' section at the back of the book gives some suggestions for organizations that may help you find experienced professionals.

Chapter 12

# Comforting Touch in End of Life Care

Comfort and quality of life are priorities as health declines. If no medical cure or improvement is possible, and an individual is approaching end of life, they may enroll on a hospice program offering palliative services that seek to provide comfort while controlling pain and managing symptoms of disease. Hospice care can be delivered at home or in a healthcare facility. It often involves an integrative approach. In addition to whatever medical treatment is necessary, palliative care also considers a person's social, spiritual and psychological needs. Conventional nursing, pastoral care and social services may be augmented by mind-body therapies, massage, aromatherapy, acupuncture or other techniques.

When someone is dying, there are a number of medications and treatments that will alleviate some of the symptoms they may experience. These include medications and treatments to help them relax, alleviate pain, resolve agitation, improve their breathing using oxygen therapy and to dry up secretions that are causing congestion. The dying phase can be a very active process. The person may experience a number of symptoms, some of which appear to be distressing and hard to observe. The dying person may be comatose or agitated, with difficulty breathing and audible chest congestion. They may have a fever and feel hot to the touch on their chest or forehead, but have cold hands and feet. Others may be resting quietly and peacefully when they take their last breaths.

When a loved one is dying, staying with the person is a priority. People need support during the dying process, especially if they have had a protracted illness. Many healthcare professionals, especially members of a hospice team, caregivers and family will start a vigil and take turns staying with the dying person. While medical treatments can aid physical comfort, caregivers may also want to contribute through their presence and touch. A hand massage can be of value to learn in advance and to share when the dying process starts. Then, if you feel compelled to touch and it feels right, you will know what to do. It can make the experience at end of life more meaningful and is often what the caregiver later remembers. The effects of touch create a special bond.

You may find that bearing witness to a person who is actively dying will affect you emotionally in ways that you may or may not expect. Remember that your presence makes a difference and that even without touching the dying person, your compassion and concern is of value. It may also feel like a gift to be afforded the opportunity to be present at such a meaningful time.

## Attending to comfort

In a hospice situation, when the goals of care focus on comfort and pain relief, touch can play an important role. The plan of care may change frequently during this time and certain previous restrictions may be eased. The hospice team works together to do whatever they can to alleviate suffering and improve quality of life.

One study compared 'massage' and 'touch' for their ability to decrease pain and distress and improve quality of life for people with advanced cancer. The 'massage' was performed by a massage therapist who chose the types of strokes and location—mostly the upper body—for about 30 minutes. The use of 'touch' involved placement of both hands on the receiver for three minutes at various locations—the neck, shoulder blades, low back, calves, heels, knees, feet, clavicles, lower arms and hands—for a total of 30 minutes. To try to eliminate the known effects of intention, the givers in the control group were told to count backwards from 100 by 7, recite nursery rhymes or plan their day's activities (Kutner *et al.* 2008).

Results showed that both massage and simple touch were associated with statistically significant improvements in immediate and sustained pain outcomes. Both groups demonstrated statistically significant improvements in physical and emotional distress and quality of life across weekly assessments. Researchers noted that although there is concern about massage safety in cancer, they found 'no statistically significant differences in adverse events or deaths among this advanced cancer population' suggesting the study as a promising model for future clinical trials in the hospice and palliative care population (Kutner *et al.* 2008, p.377).

A recent study regarding the benefits of palliative care in addition to standard treatment shows that when offered to terminally ill lung cancer patients at the time of diagnosis, they reported that they were happier, more mobile and in less pain, and they lived almost three months longer than their counterparts who received only standard treatment (Temel *et al.* 2010). While the study did not detail exactly what the palliative care treatment plan was, it speaks volumes about the value of treatments and interventions that help people to feel better.

# Do they know I'm here?

A common concern for family members when their loved one loses their ability to communicate or interact normally, is in a coma, or is approaching the end of life, is whether or not they know that their loved ones are there. It's often said in despair, 'What should I do? Should I talk to her? Does she know I'm here?' When told that, yes, they do know you are here, the sense of relief is significant and the family members often engage the comatose person further. Touch can be a helpful addition to any communication with someone who is not able to respond, since often our touch further conveys our feelings and intentions.

Sharing massage with someone who is not conscious presents challenges that require some thought. Some people may appear to be unconscious, but are able to respond by blinking an eye or by lifting a finger to communicate their wishes. People who are in an unconscious state are not able to communicate with you, respond to you, or provide feedback about the massage. If you are not responsible for the receiver's care, you must obtain permission for massage, in collaboration with the physician and healthcare team.

Before starting massage, if you are not usually involved with the receiver's hands-on care, you may need to ask other caregivers to turn and position the comatose person so that you can perform massage. The comatose person's airway and breathing must be protected, so positioning them flat on their back is not recommended. You may also need to use pillows and bolsters to support them in the best position for massage. Make sure their head is positioned so breathing is easy and once positioned, check that the bolsters and pillows are not blocking the airway or interfering with breathing.

Sharing hand massage with a person who is comatose may feel awkward and you may not think that it is helpful. Despite the comatose person's inability to communicate with you, you should feel free to talk to the person and explain what you are doing during the massage. Massage strokes should be light and applied conservatively. You may notice contractures and other effects of bed rest in addition to loss of muscle mass, tone, connective tissue and underlying fat stores if the person has been comatose for an extended period of time. If in doubt, just hold their hand with a mindful presence.

Caring for people who are no longer verbal or who are not conscious, may leave the caregiver wondering if their presence makes any difference. This question weighs heavily on family members, friends and caregivers, and was what inspired psychotherapist Jeanne Denney to create a unique study that looked at how presence might affect someone in a comatose state.

'The biofeedback program from the Institute of HeartMath seemed like a good tool to use,' Ms. Denney explained, 'because it was developed as a way to use measurable physical parameters to study non-verbal interaction and connection to emotional states.' She recruited volunteers who had some training in either meditation or bodywork of some kind, to be the 'experimental' ingredient. They were told to practice some sort of centering technique before they went into the hospice room. Then sensors were put onto the fingers of both the giver and receiver, and their heart rate variability (HRV) patterns were compared as the sitter stayed next to the patient's bedside. Could the volunteer have enough of an effect on the patient's heart rate variability to cause it to 'entrain', or mirror, their own?

'Though getting actual coherence patterns in a hospice population is rare, we did on average find increased levels of coherence, with simultaneous response patterns in HRV of both the sitter and the patient being displayed in the graphs,' Ms. Denney said. Her study, which involved four receivers, showed that they had an increase in coherence in 14 out of 28 sittings with the volunteers. In 24 decipherable sittings, simultaneous responses were noted in 23 of them (Denney 2008).

There were clear instances of the capacity to develop relationship while in a comatose state. 'For example, there was one patient in a comatose state who I had worked with for ten months prior to the study,' Ms. Denney explained. 'This patient was in a session with a sitter when I came to check on the readings; when I walked into the room, the patient's heart rate pattern changed and registered a more coherent state.' Touch, when used in some of the later sessions, initially created something like a startle reaction, which makes a case for the mindful and aware approach one should use for someone in this state.

Ms. Denney feels that this pilot study supports the experience of caregivers and people who work with the dying that a subtle exchange takes place even when people are in non-communicating states and near the end of life. 'Patients appear to need supportive relationships with regular, loving caregivers,' she concludes. 'It seems obvious that this contact would be enhanced if the caregivers understood and felt that patients were aware of them.'

Many people who are present at the time of death of a loved one talk about coincidences in timing. It has been observed that the dying person will wait for an important family member to arrive before letting go. Similarly, the dying person may seem to wait for a friend or family member to leave if they are not comfortable bearing witness to their death. Sometimes the person waits for a healthcare practitioner to be present before dying, and this is interpreted as the person's attempt to relieve family members of the responsibility for managing the situation. Often, family members are grateful to the deceased in their thoughtfulness. As evidence of the power of love, this aspect of spirit can be quite dominant in end-of-life care.

## A return to spirit

With any life changes such as illness, we wonder how it will affect our lives. There are many questions that arise. Are there important things unsaid? How do I approach the subject of dying? Are there arrangements to be made? What lies ahead? Will there be a sense of closure? People try to cope in a variety of ways.

Some caregivers are in denial, ignoring the obvious and pretending there is nothing wrong, an effective way to protect themselves from falling apart. Some may carry on with the routine of their lives because it all helps them to feel normal and remain in control. Others keep themselves distracted from thinking about their grief and the impending loss by staying busy organizing the person who is ill and getting them out of bed—sometimes against their will—for feeding, dressing and bathing.

Others express the emotions that they are feeling—fear, pain and resentment—by voicing their dissatisfaction. Many start to bargain, hoping to make changes for the better while looking for a promise of a different outcome. Most feel depressed and sad in anticipation of loss, verbalizing loneliness and unwelcome change. Finally, if the dying person seems to be suffering, their loved ones will accept the impending loss and welcome the relief that death will bring.

When there is a strong urge to keep the dying person active, massage can help to manage this urge when it is no longer practical. Spending time with the dying person doing meaningful things helps lessen the sense that time is slipping away. In the process of sharing hand massage, time seems to slow down and expand; the opportunity for conversation is realized. What are your wishes for the end of your life? How would you like us to care for you? The comfort and relaxation afforded by an intimate shared experience sets the stage for the possibility of discussion.

The touch experience can be an opportunity to reminisce about the life you have had together and do a life review. It can cover accomplishments, proud moments, big events in your lives, good times, friendships, important people, vacations and celebrations. The emotions felt at the time of the event are relived and enjoyed once again.

Maybe you will not use or need words, and enter the realm of spirit, which is the inner life you have, filled with feelings, sensations, images and dreams. This is also a flowing stream of exchange. It too can be a deeply felt sense of connection, as you slow down and forget about time. Jacques Lusseyran, a writer who was blinded as a child, described the importance of touch and its radiant nature in his book *And There Was Light*. He described sensitive touch as a way to tune into an object or person and allow the current they have to 'connect with one's own, like electricity. To put it differently, this means an end of living in front of things and a beginning of living with them' (Lusseyran 1987, p.27).

In end-of-life care, people often turn to their religious or spiritual practices for solace, support and connection to a divine source. The Reverend Jean A. Leone is executive director and administrator of Hospice and Palliative Services at Villa Marie Claire in Saddle River, NJ, a new facility developed by Holy Name Medical Center to meet the growing and critical need for compassionate end-of-life care for terminally ill patients and their loved ones. An important part of care at Villa Marie Claire is an environment where patients and families from all religious, social and economic backgrounds can feel comfortable and peaceful as they near the final stages of life's journey. It is Reverend Leone's mission to be sure that appropriate pastoral care is part of their integrative and interfaith services.

'While touch may provide comfort and connection to another human soul, it does not necessarily connect one to a "higher source",' Reverend Leone said. 'Spiritual presence in end-of-life care, I believe, is a bit different. While touch may certainly provide a stillness and initiation of connection, the importance of education and understanding within the various faith paths is needed to facilitate energy from the source, however that may be defined by the individual and their unique path.'

She explains the role of the individual providing pastoral care from an interfaith place as the ability to transcend differences and meet the individual where 'they are at'. Important to this process is providing a safe and comfortable place that allows spirit to surface and be present. 'The individual providing spiritual companionship then assists the patient or caregiver to delve into those areas of concern that may be barriers for a peaceful death,' she explained, 'such as concern about loved ones, the meaning and purpose of life, the meaning of pain and suffering, fears about death, forgiveness, questions about the "afterlife" and the individual's understanding of faith.'

As the hospice movement continues to grow, there is ever greater awareness of the need to honor whatever religious background or spiritual practices patients and their families may have. It illustrates, once again, the importance of working as a team.

# Expanding the circle of care

Caregivers, however loving they may be, are often fatigued. At home, relatives are the primary people that the dying person relies upon. They arrange and provide all the care that is needed. In the hospital or hospice, they are juggling their lives while trying to maintain their vigil. There may very well be times when they could use a massage instead of giving one.

A research study looked at the effect of a 25-minute foot or hand massage on the well-being of people providing palliative care for relatives at home. During nine sessions provided over a period of two weeks, caregivers could chose to have either a foot or hand massage. The massage was carried out with slow strokes, light pressure and circling movements, mostly done in silence. All participants had the option to receive their treatment alone or with the family member present, and most chose the latter option. They were encouraged to rest for 30 minutes after the massage session.

'Despite their worries, tiredness and burdensome situation, the massage was experienced to facilitate a sense of inner power and well-being momentarily or for an extended period of time' the researchers found (Cronfalk, Strang and Ternestedt 2009, p.2228). In interviews, all the caregivers described positive feelings, including relaxation, increased vitality and a meditative mental state.

When family members or friends ask how they can help, perhaps a hand massage to a caregiver could be a way to provide support. Creating a small group to learn and practice comforting touch with one another would offer the benefits of touch along with easing the isolation caregivers often experience. As we reach out to help, at first our individual effort seems small. But then one person extends their hand and then another. Soon there is a community of hands, helping all who take part share the radiant gift of body, energy and spirit.

## WHEN SHARING TOUCH:
## YOUR PRESENCE IS A GIFT

Robert's large, brown eyes looked sadly at his father as he lay in the nursing home bed. His father had recently returned from the hospital and he was different. He seemed less 'present', more a part of the next world than this one. At the moment he was sound asleep, lying on his back making snoring noises that cut across the room.

Robert was participating in a research project on touch and had been giving his father a hand massage over the course of a few weeks. But now he wondered if he should touch his father or leave him alone. The question of whether or not to use comforting touch on a sleeping resident had been brought up with the lead psychologist in the study, who suggested that if a resident were asleep when approached for touch, the caregivers should consider the context.

Was it just after lunch, a natural naptime for many residents? Had the resident experienced any difficulty the previous night or earlier in the day? Was the resident usually agitated and would the rest be important to their well-being? If the answer to any of these was yes, then the caregiver would either skip the session or, if possible, consider returning later. If, however, the resident was usually drifting in and out of sleep, had few visitors and hence little opportunity for touch, then the caregiver could proceed if it felt right to them.

Since Robert's father had been unconscious much of the time since his return from the hospital, Robert decided to proceed with the touch. He had the doctor's okay to resume using touch, which indicated that there was no concern about underlying problems. Robert began his session by explaining to his father what he was going to do. He proceeded gently, watchful for any signs of resistance.

Robert was a little skeptical as he began stroking his father's arm, probably wondering, as many people might, if what he was doing would make any difference. Nevertheless, he felt since he was there, why not take advantage of the opportunity to explore the possibilities this meeting provided. He had no answers, only questions.

He slowly continued, massaging the fingers, and then holding meridian points at the fingertips. Robert, a muscular man in his early forties, stood beside the bed as he applied the touch. Though he was relaxed and proceeding gently, beads of sweat formed on his face. It was winter, and the heat in his father's room was intense that day.

Robert finished the right hand and looked at his father, who had not moved during the 15 minutes of touch, nor had there been the slightest ripple of change in his face or posture. Robert wondered if he should continue, especially since going to the other side of the bed meant standing next to the radiator, which was blasting its heat into the room.

Dutifully, yet somewhat reluctantly, Robert began to walk around the foot of the bed to the other side. As he did, a most intriguing moment occurred. His father silently raised his left hand and held it out to him, without opening his eyes, closing his mouth, or changing in any other way. Robert's big eyes grew even bigger as he took that in with astonishment. The research could not capture this event; it was not set up to tell the individual stories. Yet, here was one of the profound experiences that made this kind of project so rewarding. It was also a lesson to remind us that we do not have to journey to remote places to confront the unknown; our own body, energy and consciousness—with us on a daily basis—offer plenty of mystery to explore.

In a non-waking state, Robert's father had used a gesture to communicate. It was as if some part of his father was saying, 'Yes, here is my hand, take my hand, and please share your enlivening touch with me. I am here, waiting for you.' Robert went to the other side of the bed and took his father's hand, now with a little more confidence that presence and touch were being shared by them both.

## THE INNER PRACTICE: ENDING A SESSION

When you feel you have reached the end of the time for sharing comforting touch, create a sense of completion by following some closing steps. Having predictable ways of beginning and ending will communicate your intention to the receiver and build trust with repeated use.

A simple ritual involves ending the way you began.

1. When you finish stroking the hand and arm, or holding the last meridian point, remove your hands mindfully from the physical and energetic contact. Thank the receiver for the shared time.

2. Remain beside the receiver to observe: evaluate the expression on his or her face, the rhythm of their breath, the position of their arms and hands, their disposition. Reflect on any changes you may see. Think about what you did and what you might do differently next time.

3. Observe yourself and evaluate your own breathing pattern, the physical and energetic state of your body, and thought patterns. Is there any difference now compared to when you began? Give yourself a few moments to sense and feel changes that may have occurred.

4. When you are ready, get up and go to the sink to thoroughly wash your hands. Do so mindfully, letting the water be a source of cleansing and at the same time a sense of connection to the renewing energies of nature.

# Resources

## AGING AND DEMENTIA

### Australia

Department of Health and Ageing
Sirius Building, Furzer Street
Woden Town Centre
GPO Box 9848
Canberra ACT 2601
Phone: 02 6289 1555
Website: www.health.gov.au

Alzheimer's Australia
1 Frewin Place
Scullin ACT
Phone: 02 6254 4233
Fax: 02 6278 7225
Hotline: 1 800 100 500
Email: nat.admin@alzheimers.org.au
Website: www.alzheimers.org.au

### Canada

Health Canada
Address Locator 0900C2
Ottawa, Ontario K1A 0K9
Phone: 613 957 2991
Fax: 613 941 5366
Email: Info@hc-sc.gc.ca
Website: www.hc-sc.gc.ca

Alzheimer Society of Canada
20 Eglinton Ave. W., Ste. 1600
Toronto, ON M4R 1K8
Phone: 416 488 8772
Toll-free: 1 800 616 8816 (valid
only in Canada)
Fax: 416 322 6656
Email: info@alzheimer.ca
Website: www.alzheimer.ca

### United Kingdom

Alzheimer's Society
Devon House, 58 St Katharine's
Way
London E1W 1LB
Phone: 020 7423 3500
Fax: 020 7423 3501
Email: enquiries@alzheimers.org.uk
Website: www.alzheimers.org.uk

Age UK, National Offices:

England
Tavis House
1-6 Tavistock Square
London WC1H 9NA
Phone: 0800 169 8787
Email: contact@ageuk.org.uk
Website: www.ageuk.org.uk

Northern Ireland
3 Lower Crescent
Belfast BT7 1NR
Phone: 028 9024 5729
Email: info@ageni.org
Website: www.ageuk.org.uk

Scotland
Causewayside House
160 Causewayside
Edinburgh EH9 1PR
Phone: 0845 125 9732
Email: enquiries@
ageconcernandhelptheagedscotland.
org.uk
Website: www.ageuk.org.uk

Wales
Ty^ John Pathy
13/14 Neptune Court, Vanguard
Way
Cardiff CF24 5PJ
Phone: 029 2043 1555
Email: enquiries@agecymru.org.uk
Website: www.ageuk.org.uk

## United States

Administration on Aging
One Massachusetts Avenue NW
Washington, DC 20001
Phone: 202 619 0724
Fax: 202 357 3555
Email: aoainfo@aoa.hhs.gov
Website: www.aoa.gov

Aging with Dignity
PO Box 1661
Tallahassee, FL 32302-1661
Phone: 850 681 2010
Toll-free: 888 594 7437
Fax: 850 681 2481
Email: fivewishes@
agingwithdignity.org
Website: www.agingwithdignity.org

Alzheimer's Foundation of America
322 8th Ave., 7th Fl.
New York, NY 10001
Phone: 866 232 8484
Fax: 646 638 1546
Website: www.alzfdn.org

Center for Medicare & Medicaid
Services
7500 Security Boulevard
Baltimore, MD 21244
Phone: 877 486 2048
Toll-free: 800 633 4227
Website: www.cms.gov

National Health Council
1730 M Street NW, Suite 500
Washington, DC 20036-4561
Phone: 202 785 3910
Fax: 202 785 5923
Website: www.nhcouncil.org

National Institute on Aging
Building 31, Room 5C27
31 Center Drive, MSC 2292
Bethesda, MD 20892
Phone: 301 496 1752
Toll-free: 800 222 4225
Fax: 301 496 1072
Website: www.nia.nih.gov

# CAREGIVERS
## Australia
Department of Families, Housing, Community Services and Indigenous Affairs
Tuggeranong Office Park
Soward Way
Greenway ACT 2900
PO Box 7576
Canberra Business Centre ACT 2610
Phone: 1300 653 227
Email: enquiries@fahcsia.gov.au
Website: www.fahcsia.gov.au/sa/carers

## Canada
Alzheimer's Foundation for Caregiving in Canada
95 Mural Street, Suite 600
Richmond Hill
Ontario L4B 3G2
Toll-free: 1 877 321 2594
Phone: 905 882 3141
Fax: 905.882.3132
Email: info@alzfdn.ca
Website: www.alzfdn.ca

Canadian Caregiver Coalition
Email: ccc@ccc-ccan.ca
Website: www.ccc-ccan.ca

Family Caregivers' Network Society
526 Michigan Street
Victoria, BC V8V 1S2
Phone: 250 384 0408
Toll-free: 1 877 520 FCNS (3267) within British Columbia
Fax: 250 361 2660
Email: fcns@telus.net
Website: www.fcns-caregiving.org

Service Canada
Canada Enquiry Centre
Ottawa, ON K1A 0J9
Toll-free: 1 800 O-Canada (1 800 622 6232)
Website: www.servicecanada.gc.ca/eng/lifeevents/caregiver.shtml

## United Kingdom
Carers UK, Regional Offices:

Carers UK
20 Great Dover Street
London SE1 4LX
Phone: 020 7378 4999
Website: www.carersuk.org

Carers Northern Ireland
58 Howard Street
Belfast BT1 6JP
Phone: 02890 439 843
Website: www.carersuk.org

Carers Scotland
The Cottage
21 Pearce Street
Glasgow G51 3UT
Phone: 0141 445 3070
Website: www.carersuk.org

Carers Wales
River House
Ynys Bridge Court
Cardiff CF15 9SS
Phone: 02920 811 370
Website: www.carersuk.org

The Princess Royal Trust for Carers,
Regional Offices:
Glasgow Office
Charles Oakley House
125 West Regent Street
Glasgow G2 2SD
Phone: 0141 221 5066
Fax: 0141 221 4623
Email: info@carers.org
Website: www.carers.org

London Office
Unit 14, Bourne Court
Southend Road
Woodford Green
Essex IG8 8HD
Phone: 0844 800 4361
Fax: 0844 800 4362
Email: info@carers.org
Website: www.carers.org

Wales Office
Victoria House
250 Cowbridge Road East
Canton
Cardiff CF5 1GZ
Phone: 02920 221788
Email: info@carers.org
Website: www.carers.org

## United States
National Family Caregivers
Association
10400 Connecticut Avenue, Suite 500
Kensington, MD 20895-3944
Phone: 301 942 6430
Toll-free: 800 896 3650
Fax: 301 942 2302
Email: info@thefamilycaregiver.org
Website: www.nfcacares.org

National Alliance for Caregiving
4720 Montgomery Lane, 2nd Floor
Bethesda, MD 20814
Phone: 301 718 8444
Website: www.caregiving.org/contact-us

# GENERAL
## International
World Health Organization
Avenue Appia 20
1211 Geneva 27, Switzerland
Phone: 22 791 21 11
Fax: 22 791 31 11
Email: info@who.int
Website: www.who.int/en

## United Kingdom
Evidence in Health and Social Care
Phone: 0845 003 77 44
Email: contactus@evidence.nhs.uk
Website: www.evidence.nhs.uk

National Institute for Health
Research
Richmond House
Room 132
79 Whitehall
London SW1A 2NS
Email: enquiries@nihr.ac.uk
Website: www.nihr.ac.uk

## United States
Center for Disease Control and
Prevention
1600 Clifton Rd
Atlanta, GA 30333
Phone: 800 232 4636
Email: cdcinfo@cdc.gov
Website: www.cdc.gov

# HOSPICE AND PALLIATIVE CARE

## Australia

CareSearch Palliative Care
Knowledge Network
Palliative Care Knowledge Network
Project
Health Sciences Building
Repatriation General Hospital
Daws Road
Daw Park, SA 5041
Phone: 08 7221 8233 (within
Australia)
Phone: +618 7221 8233
(international callers)
Fax: 08 7221 8238
Email: caresearch@flinders.edu.au
Website: www.caresearch.com.au

Palliative Care Australia
Suite 4, 37 Geils Court
Deakin, ACT 2600
Phone: 02 6232 4433
Fax: 02 6232 4434
Email: pcainc@palliativecare.org.au
Website: www.palliativecare.org.au

## Canada

Canadian Hospice Palliative Care
Association
Annex D, Saint-Vincent Hospital
60 Cambridge Street North
Ottawa, ON K1R 7A5
Phone: 613 241 3663
Toll-free: 800 668 2785
Fax: 613 241 3986
Email: info@chpca.net
Website: www.chpca.net

Canadian Virtual Hospice
Room PE469, One Morley Avenue
Winnipeg, MB R3L 2P4
Email: info@virtualhospice.ca
Website: www.virtualhospice.ca

Hospice Association of Ontario
2 Carlton Street, Suite 707
Toronto, ON M5B 1J3
Phone: 416 304 1477
Toll-free: 800 349 3111
Fax: 416 304 1479
Email: info@hospice.on.ca
Website: www.hospice.on.ca

## International

International Association for the
Study of Pain
IASP Secretariat
111 Queen Anne Ave N, Suite 501
Seattle, WA 98109-4955 USA
Phone: 206 283 0311
Fax: 206 283 9403
Email: IASPdesk@iasp-pain.org
Website: www.iasp-pain.org

## United Kingdom

Help the Hospices
Hospice House
34-44 Britannia Street
London WC1X 9JG
Phone: 020 7520 8200
Fax: 020 7278 1021
Email: info@helpthehospices.org.uk
Website: www.helpthehospices.org.uk

The National Council for Palliative Care
The Fitzpatrick Building
188–194 York Way
London N7 9AS
Phone: 020 7697 1520
Fax: 020 7697 1530
Email: enquiries@ncpc.org.uk
Website: www.ncpc.org.uk

## United States

American Academy of Hospice and Palliative Medicine
4700 W. Lake Avenue
Glenview, IL 60025-1485
Phone: 847 375 4712
Fax: 847 375 6475
Email: info@aahpm.org
Website: www.aahpm.org

Center to Advance Palliative Care
1255 Fifth Avenue, Suite C-2
New York, NY 10029
Phone: 212 201 2670
Email: capc@mssm.edu
Website: www.capc.org

Mount Sinai Medical Center
The Hertzberg Palliative Care Institute
One Gustav I. Levy Place
PO Box 1070
New York, NY 10029
Phone: 212 241 1446
Fax: 212 426 5054
www.mountsinai.org/patient-care

National Hospice and Palliative Care Organization
1731 King Street, Suite 100
Alexandria, VA 22314
Phone: 703 837 1500
Fax: 703 837 1233
Email: nhpco_info@nhpco.org
Website: www.nhpco.org

National Hospice Foundation
1731 King Street, Suite 200
Alexandria, VA 22314
Phone: 877 470 6472
Email: info@
nationalhospicefoundation.org
Website: www.
nationalhospicefoundation.org

Practitioner Solutions
Phone: 212 517 1775
Email: info@practitionersolutions.com
Website: www.practitionersolutions.com

Villa Marie Claire
Hospice and Palliative Services
12 West Saddle River Road
Saddle River, NJ 07458
Phone: 201 833 3188
Toll-free: 1 866 979 7787
Fax: 201 833 3164
Email: vmc@holyname.org

# INTEGRATIVE CARE
## Canada
Canadian Interdisciplinary Network
for Complementary and Alternative
Medicine Research
University of Calgary
Faculty of Medicine
Department of Community Health
Services
3280 Hospital Drive, NW
Calgary, AB T2 4Z6
Phone: 403 270 7307
Fax: 403 270 7307
Email: akania@ucalgary.ca
Website: www.incamresearch.ca

## United Kingdom
BioMed Central
236 Gray's Inn Road
London WC1X 8HB
Email: info@biomedcentral.com
Website: www.biomedcentral.com

Complementary & Natural
Healthcare Council
83 Victoria Street
London SW1H 0HW
Phone: 020 3178 2199
Email: info@cnhc.org.uk
Website: http://cnhc.org.uk

## United States
Bravewell Collaborative
1818 Oliver Ave. South
Minneapolis, MN 55405
Email: info@bravewell.org
Website: www.bravewell.org

Center for Mindfulness in Medicine,
Health Care and Society
University of Massachusetts Medical
School
Chang Building
222 Maple Ave.
Shrewsbury, MA 01545
Mailing address:
55 Lake Avenue North
Worcester, MA 01655
Phone: 508 856 2656
Fax: 508 856 1977
Email: mindfulness@umassmed.edu
Website: www.umassmed.edu

Institute of HeartMath
14700 W. Park Avenue
Boulder Creek, CA 95006
Phone: 831.338.8500
Toll-free: 800 711 6221
Fax: 831 338 8504
Email: info@heartmath.org
Website: www.heartmath.org

Memorial Sloan-Kettering Cancer
Center
Integrative Medicine Services
Outpatient: The Bendheim
Integrative Medicine Center
1429 First Avenue
New York, NY 10065
Inpatient: Memorial Sloan-Kettering
Cancer Center
1275 York Avenue
New York, NY 10065
Phone: 646 888 0800
Website for Integrative Services:
www.mskcc.org/mskcc/html/1979.
cfm
Website for herbs, botanicals and
other products: www.mskcc.org/
mskcc/html/11570.cfm

Morgan Stanley Children's Hospital of New York-Presbyterian Integrative Therapies for Children with Cancer
3959 Broadway
New York, NY 10032
Phone: 212 342 8579
Website: http://childrensnyp.org/mschony/patients/for-visitors/integrative-therapies.html

National Center for Complementary and Alternative Medicine
NCCAM Clearinghouse
PO Box 7923
Gaithersburg, MD 20898
Phone: 1 888 644 6226
Fax: 1 866 464 3616
Email: info@nccam.nih.gov
Website: www.nccam.nih.gov

Samueli Institute
1737 King Street, Suite 600
Alexandria, VA 22314
Phone: 703 299 4800
Website: www.siib.org

Society for Integrative Oncology
(No street address available)
Phone: 646 504 4SIO (4746)
Website: www.integrativeonc.org

School of Images
73 Fifth Avenue
New York, NY 10003
Phone: 212 627 5904
Email: info@schoolofimages.com
Website: www.schoolofimages.com

St. Joseph's Hospital for Children
703 Main Street
Paterson, NJ 07503
Phone: 973 754 2500
Website: www.stjosephshealth.org

# MASSAGE THERAPY AND SHIATSU

Professional organizations that provide standards of education and follow guidelines usually have a search function for members who meet the qualifications for practice. Local accredited schools may also be a source for finding practitioners.

## Australia

Australian Association of Massage Therapists
Level 6, 85 Queen St, Melbourne VIC 3000
Phone: 1300 138 872 or 03 9691 3700
Fax: 03 9602 3088
Email: info@aamt.com.au
Website: www.aamt.com.au

Australian Acupuncture and Chinese Medical Association
PO Box 1635
Coorparoo DC, QLD 4151
Phone: 07 3324 2599
Fax: 07 3394 2399
Email: aacma@acupuncture.org.au
Website: www.acupuncture.org.au

Shiatsu Therapy Association of Australia
PO Box 248
Surrey Hills, VIC 3127
Phone: 1300 138 250
Fax 03 9890 5701
Email: enquiries@staa.org.au
Website: www.staa.org.au

## Canada

Massage Therapy Alliance of
Canada
581 Huron Street
Toronto, ON
M5R 2R6
Phone: 416 929 9759
Email: info@massage.ca
Website: http://massage.ca

## United Kingdom

Academy of Classical Chinese
Medicine (Ireland)
1 Summerhill Parade
Sandycove, Co Dublin
Phone/Fax: +353 1 2801950
Email: summerhillclinic@eircom.net
Website: www.accm.ie

British Acupuncture Council
63 Jeddo Road
London W12 9HQ
Phone: 020 8735 0400
Fax: 020 8735 0404
Website: www.acupuncture.org.uk

General Council for Massage
Therapies
27 Old Gloucester Street
London WC1N 3XX
Phone: 0870 850 4452
Email: gcmt@btconnect.com
Website: http://gcmt.org.uk

Shiatsu Society (UK)
PO Box 4580
Rugby
Warwickshire CV21 9EL
Phone: 0845 130 4560
Fax: 01788 547111
Website: www.shiatsusociety.org

## United States

American Association of
Acupuncture and Oriental Medicine
PO Box 162340
Sacramento, CA 95816
Phone: 866 455 7999
Fax: 916 443 4766
Website: www.aaaomonline.org

American Massage Therapy
Association
500 Davis Street, Suite 900
Evanston, IL 60201-4695
Phone: 877 905 0577
Fax: 847 864 5196
Email: info@amtamassage.org
Website: www.amtamassage.org

American Organization for
Bodywork Therapies of Asia
1010 Haddonfield-Berlin Road,
Suite 408
Voorhees, NJ 0804203-3514
Phone: 856 782 1616
Fax: 856 782 1653
Email: office@aobta.org
Website: www.aobta.org

National Certification Board for
Therapeutic Massage and Bodywork
1901 South Meyers Road, Suite
240
Oakbrook Terrace, IL 60181
Phone: 630 627 8000
Email: info@ncbtmb.org
Website: www.ncbtmb.org

Touch Research Institutes
University of Miami School of
Medicine
Mailman Center for Child
Development
1601 NW 12th Ave., 7th Floor,
Suite 7037
Miami, FL 33101
Phone: 305 243 6781
Fax: 305 243 6488
Email: tfield@med.miami.edu
Website: www6.miami.edu/touch-
research/About.html

# References

Alexander, W. (2009) 'HeartMath.' *Lilipoh 14*, 55. Accessed on May 26, 2011 at www.lilipoh.com/articles/2009Issues/Spring2009/HeartMath.aspx

Bakalar, N. (2009) 'Five-second touch can convey specific emotion, study finds.' *New York Times*, August 11, 2009, p.D3.

Barnett, K. (1972) 'A survey of the current utilization of touch by health team personnel with hospitalized patients.' *International Journal of Nursing Studies 9*, 4, 195–209.

Benjamin, B.E. and Sohnen-Moe, C. (2005) *The Ethics of Touch*. Tucson, AZ: SMA Inc.

Broyard, A. (1990) 'Good books about being sick' [Book review]. *New York Times*, April 1, 29.

Butts, J.B. (2001) 'Outcomes of comfort touch in institutionalized elderly female patients.' *Geriatric Nursing 22*, 4, 180–184.

Cassileth, B.R. and Vickers, A.J. (2004) 'Massage therapy for symptom control: Outcome study at a major cancer center.' *Journal of Pain and Symptom Management 28*, 3, 244–249.

Center for Disease Control and Prevention (2010) *Hand Hygiene Basics*. Atlanta, GA: Center for Disease Control and Prevention. Accessed on May 26, 2011 at www.cdc.gov/handhygiene/Basics.html

Chao, L.F., Zhang, A.L., Liu, H.E., Cheng, M.H., Lam H.B. and Lo, S.K. (2009) 'The efficacy of acupoint stimulation for the management of therapy-related adverse events in patients with breast cancer: A systematic review.' *Breast Cancer Research and Treatment 118*, 2, 255–267.

Chen, M.L., Lin L.C., Wu S.C., Lin, J.G. (1999) 'The effectiveness of acupressure in improving the quality of sleep of institutionalized residents.' *The Journals of Gerontology Series A: Biological Sciences and Medical Sciences 54*, 8, 389–394.

Childre, D. and Martin, H. (with Beech, D.) (2000) *The HeartMath Solution*. San Francisco, CA: HarperSanFrancisco.

Cleary, T. (trans.) (1986) *The Inner Teachings of Taoism by Chang Po-Tuan*. Boston, MA: Shambhala Publications.

Clement, J. (1987) 'Touch: Research findings and use in preoperative care.' *AORN Journal 45*, 6, 1429–1439.

Coakley, A.B. and Duffy, M.E. (2010) 'The effect of therapeutic touch on postoperative patients.' *Journal of Holistic Nursing 28*, 3, 193–200.

Cronfalk, B.S., Strang, P. and Ternestedt, B.M. (2009) 'Inner power, physical strength and existential well-being in daily life: Relatives' experiences of receiving soft tissue massage in palliative home care.' *Journal of Clinical Nursing 18*, 15, 2225–2233.

Denney, J. (2008) 'The effects of compassionate presence on people in comatose states near death.' *United States Association for Body Psychotherapy Journal 7*, 2, 11–25.

Eisenberg, D.M., Kessler, R.C., Foster, C., Norlock, F.E., Calkins, D.R. and Delbanco, T.L. (1993) 'Unconventional medicine in the United States. Prevalence, costs, and patterns of use.' *New England Journal of Medicine 328*, 4, 246–252.

Ellis, A., Wiseman, N. and Boss, K. (1991) *Fundamentals of Chinese Acupuncture* (revised edn). Brookline, MA: Paradigm Publications.

Field, T (2000) *Touch Therapy*. London: Churchill Livingstone.

Field, T.M., Schanberg, S.M., Scafidi, F. Bauer, C.R., Vega-Lahr, V., Garcia, R., Nystrom, J. and Kuhn, C.M. (1986) 'Tactile/kinesthetic stimulation effects on preterm neonates.' *Pediatrics 77*, 5, 654–658.

Gallob, R. (2003) 'Reiki: A supportive therapy in nursing practice and self-care for nurses.' *Journal of New York State Nurses Association 34*, 1, 9–13.

Gray, H. (1977) *Anatomy, Descriptive and Surgical.* Revised American, from the fifteenth English, edition (Pick, T.P. and Howden, R., eds). New York, NY: Bounty Books.

Harris, M. and Richards, K.C. (2010) 'Physiological and psychological effects of slow-stroke back massage and hand massage on relaxation in older people.' *Journal of Clinical Nursing 19*, 7–8, 917–926.

Hawranik, P., Johnston, P. and Deatrich, J. 'Therapeutic Touch and Agitation in Individuals with Alzheimer's Disease.' *Western Journal of Nursing Research, 30*, 4, 417–434.

Hertenstein, M.J., Keltner, D., App, B., Bulleit, B.A. and Jaskolka, A.R. (2006) 'Touch communicates distinct emotions.' *Emotion 6*, 3, 528–533.

Hertenstein, M.J., Holmes, R., McCullough, M. and Keltner, D. (2009) 'The communication of emotion via touch.' *Emotion 9*, 4, 566–573.

Hicks-Moore, S.L. and Robinson, B.A. (2008) 'Two interventions to decrease agitation in residents with dementia.' *Dementia: The International Journal of Social Research and Practice 7*, 1, 95–108.

Hollinger, L.M. and Buschmann, M.B.T. (1993) 'Factors influencing the perception of touch by elderly nursing home residents and their health caregivers.' *International Journal of Nursing Studies 30*, 5, 445–461.

Hsieh, L.L., Kuo, C.H., Lee, L.H., Yen, A.M., Chien, K.L. and Chen, T.H. (2006) 'Treatment of low back pain by acupressure and physical therapy: Randomised controlled trial.' *British Medical Journal 332*, 7543, 696–700. doi:10.1136/bmj.38744.672616.AE. Accessed on May 26, 2011 at www.ncbi.nlm.nih.gov/pmc/articles/PMC1410852

Institute of HeartMath (2011) *Welcome to Tools for Well-Being.* Accessed on May 7, 2011 at www.heartmath.org/free-services/tools-for-well-being/tools-for-well-being-home.html

International Center for Reiki Training (2011) *What is Reiki?* Southfield, MI: International Center for Reiki Training. Accessed on April 29, 2011 at www.reiki.org/faq/whatisreiki.html

Jhaveri, A., Walsh, S.J., Wang, Y., McCarthy, M. and Gronowicz, G. (2008) 'Therapeutic touch affects DNA synthesis and mineralization of human osteoblasts in culture.' *Journal of Orthopaedic Research 26*, 11, 1541–1546.

Kaada, B. and Torsteinbø, O. (1989) 'Increase of plasma ß-endorphins in connective tissue massage.' *General Pharmacology: The Vascular System 20*, 4, 487–489.

Kilstoff, K. and Chenoweth, L. (1998) 'New approaches to health and well-being for dementia day-care clients, family carers and day-care staff.' *International Journal of Nursing Practice 4*, 70–83.

Kim, M.S., Cho, K.S., Woo, H.M. and Kim, J.H. (2001) 'Effects of hand massage on anxiety in cataract surgery using local anesthesia.' *Journal of Cataract & Refractive Surgery 27*, 6, 884–890.

Kolcaba, K., Schirm, V. and Steiner, R. (2006) 'Effects of hand massage on comfort of nursing home residents.' *Geriatric Nursing 27*, 2, 85–91.

Kramer, N. and Smith, M. (1999) 'Music and touch therapies for nursing home residents with severe dementia.' *LTC: Psychologists in Long Term Care Newsletter 12*, 4, 7–8.

Kutner, J.S., Smith, M.C., Corbin, L., Hemphill, L., Benton, K., Mellis, B.K., Beaty, B., Felton, S., Yamashita, T.E., Bryant, L.L. and Fairclough, D.L. (2008) 'Massage therapy versus simple touch to improve pain and mood in patients with advanced cancer.' *Annals of Internal Medicine 149*, 6, 369–379.

Labyak, S.E. and Metzger, B.L. (1997) 'The effects of effleurage backrub on the physiological components of relaxation: A meta-analysis.' *Nursing Research 46*, 1, 59–62.

Leboyer, F. (1976) *Loving Hands: The Traditional Art of Baby Massage.* New York, NY: Newmarket Press.

Lee, M.S., Pittler, M.H. and Ernst, E. (2008) 'Effects of Reiki in clinical practice: A systematic review of randomized clinical trials'. *International Journal of Clinical Practice 62*, 6, 947–954.

Long, A.F. (2008) 'The effectiveness of Shiatsu: Findings from a cross-European, prospective observational study.' Journal of Alternative and Complementary Medicine 14, 8, 921–930.

Lowen, A. (1990) Bioenergetics for Grace and Harmony. New York, NY: Macmillan.

Lusseyran, J. (1987) And There Was Light. New York, NY: Parabola Books.

Maciocia, G. (1989) The Foundations of Chinese Medicine: A Comprehensive Text for Acupuncturists and Herbalists. London: Churchill Livingston.

Malaquin-Pavan, E. (1997) 'Therapeutic benefit of touch-massage in the overall management of demented elderly.' Recherche en Soins Infirmiers 49, 11–66.

Matsubara, T., Arai, Y.C., Shiro, Y., Shimo, K., Nishihara, M., Sato, J. and Ushida, T. (2011) 'Comparative effects of acupressure at local and distal acupuncture points on pain conditions and autonomic function in females with chronic neck pain.' Hindawi Publishing Corporation, Evidence-Based Complementary and Alternative Medicine, vol. 2011, article ID 543291, 6 pages. doi: 10.1155/2011/543291. Accessed on May 26, 2011 at www.hindawi.com/journals/ecam/2011/543291

McCraty, R., Atkinson, M., Tomasino, D. and Tiller, W.A. (1998) 'The Electricity of Touch: Detection and Measurement of Cardiac Energy Exchange Between People.' In K.H. Pribram (ed) Brain and Values: Is a Biological Science of Values Possible? Mahwah, NJ: Lawrence Erlbaum Associates. Available at www.heartmath.org/research/research-publications/electricity-of-touch-page-7.html

Memorial Sloan-Kettering Cancer Center (2011) Integrative Medicine Service. New York, NY: Memorial Sloan-Kettering Cancer Center. Accessed on May 9, 2011 at www.mskcc.org/mskcc/html/1979.cfm

Montagu, A. (1978) Touching: The Human Significance of the Skin (2nd edn). New York, NY: Harper & Row.

Moore, J.R. and Gilbert, D.A. (1995) 'Elderly residents: Perceptions of nurses' comforting touch.' Journal of Gerontological Nursing 21, 1, 6–13.

Mower, M. (1999) 'Massage boosts the immune system.' Massage Magazine, March/April, 50–54.

Moyer C.A., Rounds J. and Hannum, J.W. (2004) 'A meta-analysis of massage therapy research.' Psychological Bulletin 130, 1, 3–18.

New York State Office of the Professions (2010) Education Law, Article 155, Massage Therapy. New York, NY: New York State Education Department. Accessed on April 28, 2011 at www.op.nysed.gov/prof/mt/article155.htm

Ni, M. (trans) (1995) The Yellow Emperor's Classic of Medicine: A New Translation of the Neijing Suwen with Commentary. Boston, MA: Shambhala Publications.

Oh, H.J. and Park, J.S. (2004) 'Effects of hand massage and hand holding on the anxiety in patients with local infiltration anesthesia.' Taehan Kanho Hakhoe Chi 34, 6, 924–933.

Olson, K. and Hanson, J. (1997) 'Using Reiki to manage pain: A preliminary report.' Cancer Prevention and Control 1, 2, 108–113.

Osaka, I., Kurihara, V., Tanaka, K., Nishizaki, H., Aoki, S. and Adachi, I. (2009) 'Endocrinological evaluations of brief hand massages in palliative care.' Journal of Alternative and Complementary Medicine 15, 9, 981–985.

Oschman, J. (2000) Energy Medicine: The Scientific Basis. London: Churchill Livingston.

Pearce, J.C. (1980) Magical Child: Rediscovering Nature's Plan for Our Children. New York, NY: Bantam Books.

Pearce, L. (2010) 'What is Therapeutic Touch?' Therapeutic Touch Network of Canada (TTNO) newsletter, in touch, Autumn 2010. Accessed on April 18, 2011 at www.therapeutictouchontario.org/index.php/newsletter/articles-therapeutictouch/whatistherapeutictouch

Rapaport, M.H., Schettler, P. and Bresee, C. (2010) 'A preliminary study of the effects of a single session of Swedish massage on hypothalamic-pituitary-adrenal and immune function in normal individuals.' Journal of Alternative and Complementary Medicine 16, 10, 1079–1088.

Remington, R. (2002) 'Calming music and hand massage with agitated elderly.' *Nursing Research* 51, 5, 317–323.

Robert H. Lurie Comprehensive Cancer Center of Northwestern University (2004) *Introduction to Goals of Care*. Accessed on May 26, 2011 at http://endoflife.northwestern.edu/goals_of_care/what.cfm#A Brief Introduction

Sansone, P. and Schmitt, L. (2000) 'Providing tender touch massage to elderly nursing home residents: A demonstration project.' *Geriatric Nursing 21*, 6, 303–308.

Shainberg, C. (2005) *Kabbalah and the Power of Dreaming*. Rochester, VT: Inner Traditions.

Smith, A., Kimmel, S. and Milz, S. (2010) 'Effects of therapeutic touch on pain, function and well being in persons with osteo-arthritis of the knee: A pilot study.' *Internet Journal of Advanced Nursing Practice 10*, 2, 1–25. Accessed on May 9, 2011 at www.ispub.com/journal/the_internet_journal_of_advanced_nursing_practice/volume_10_number_2_11/article/effects-of-therapeutic-touch-on-pain-function-and-well-being-in-persons-with-osteo-arthritis-of-the-knee-a-pilot-study.html

Snyder, M., Egan, E.C. and Burns, K.R. (1995) 'Interventions for decreasing agitation behaviors in persons with dementia.' *Journal of Gerontological Nursing 21*, 7, 34–40.

Tappan, F. and Benjamin, P. (1998) *Tappan's Handbook of Healing Massage Techniques: Classic, Holistic, and Emerging Methods* (3rd edn). Stamford, CT: Appleton & Lange.

Temel, J.S., Greer, J.A., Muzikansky, A., Gallagher, E.R., Admane, S., Jackson, V.A., Dahlin, C.M., Blinderman, C.D., Jacobsen, J., Pirl, W.F., Billings, J.A. and Lynch, T.J. (2010) 'Early palliative care for patients with metastatic non-small-cell lung cancer.' *New England Journal of Medicine 363*, 8, 733–742.

Trombley, J. (2003) 'Massage therapy for elder residents: Examining the power of touch on pain, anxiety, and strength building.' *Nursing Homes Magazine*, October 1. Accessed on May 9, 2011 at www.allbusiness.com/health-care-social-assistance/nursing/684317-1.html

Trungpa, C. (2009) *Smile at Fear: Awakening the True Heart of Bravery*. Boston, MA: Shambhala Publications.

Tsang, K.L., Carlson, L.E. and Olson, K. (2007) 'Pilot crossover trial of Reiki versus rest for treating cancer-related fatigue.' *Integrative Cancer Therapies 6*, 1, 25–35.

Uvnäs-Moberg, K. (2003) *The Oxytocin Factor: Tapping the Hormone of Calm, Love and Healing*. Cambridge, MA: Da Capo Press.

Vortherms, R. (1991) 'Clinically improving communication through touch.' *Journal of Gerontological Nursing 17*, 5, 6–9.

Wang, H.L. and Keck, J.F. (2004) 'Foot and hand massage as an intervention for postoperative pain.' *Pain Management Nursing 5*, 2, 59–65.

Wilkinson, S., Barnes, K. and Storey, L. (2008) 'Massage for symptom relief in patients with cancer: Systematic review.' *Journal of Advanced Nursing 63*, 5, 430–439.

Wong-Baker FACES Foundation (2011) 'Wong-Baker FACES Pain Rating Scale.' Accessed on June 15, 2011 at www.wongbakerfaces.org

Woods, D.L., Beck, C. and Sinha, K. (2009) 'The effect of therapeutic touch on behavioral symptoms and cortisol in persons with dementia.' *Research in Complementary Medicine 16*, 3, 181–189.

World Health Organization (2009a) *How to Handrub?* Geneva: World Health Organization. Accessed on April 10, 2011 at www.who.int/gpsc/5may/How_To_HandRub_Poster.pdf

World Health Organization (2009b) *How to Handwash?* Geneva: World Health Organization. Accessed on April 10, 2011 at www.who.int/gpsc/5may/How_To_HandWash_Poster.pdf

Yang, M.H., Wu, S.C., Lin, J.G., Lin, L.C. (2007) 'The efficacy of acupressure for decreasing agitated behavior in dementia: A pilot study.' *Journal of Clinical Nursing 16*, 2, 308–315.

Zick, S.M., Alrawi, S., Merel, G., Burris, B., Sen, A., Litzinger, A. and Harris, R.E. (2011) 'Relaxation acupressure reduces persistent cancer-related fatigue.' Hindawi Publishing Corporation, *Evidence-Based Complementary and Alternative Medicine 10, vol. 2011*, article ID 142931, 10 pages. doi: 10.1155/2011/142913. Accessed on April 15, 2011 at www.hindawi.com/journals/ecam/2011/142913/abs

# Index